THE WAISTLINE PLAN

1　　2　　3　　4　　5　　6　　7　　8　　9　　10　　11　　12　　13

hamlyn

THE WAISTLINE PLAN

BEAT MIDDLE-AGE SPREAD IN JUST 6 WEEKS!

14 15 16 17 18 19 20 21 22 23 24 25 26

Sally Lewis

Notes

It is advisable to check with your doctor before embarking on any exercise program. This book is not intended as a substitute for personal medical advice. The reader should consult a doctor in all matters relating to health and particularly in respect of any symptoms that may require diagnosis or medical attention. While the advice and information are believed to be accurate and true at the time of going to press, neither the author nor the publisher can accept any legal responsibility or liability for errors or omissions that may be made.

Ovens should be preheated to the specified temperature —if using a fan-assisted oven, follow the manufacturer's instructions for adjusting the time and the temperature.

Fresh herbs should be used unless otherwise stated.

Medium eggs should be used unless otherwise stated.

The Department of Health advises that eggs should not be consumed raw. This book contains some dishes made with raw or lightly cooked eggs. It is prudent for vulnerable people such as pregnant and nursing mothers, invalids, the elderly, babies and young children to avoid uncooked or lightly cooked dishes made with eggs. Once prepared, these dishes should be kept refrigerated and used promptly.

This book includes dishes made with nuts and nut derivatives. It is advisable for those with known allergic reactions to nuts and nut derivatives and those who may be potentially vulnerable to these allergies, such as pregnant and nursing mothers, invalids, the elderly, babies and children, to avoid dishes made with nuts and nut oils. It is also prudent to check the labels of pre-prepared ingredients for the possible inclusion of nut derivatives.

1   2   3   4   5   6   7   8   9   10   11   12   13

First published in Great Britain in 2007 by Hamlyn,
a division of Octopus Publishing Group Ltd
2–4 Heron Quays, London E14 4JP

Copyright © Octopus Publishing Group Ltd 2007

Distributed in the United States and Canada by Sterling Publishing Co., Inc., 387 Park Avenue South, New York, NY 10016–8810

ISBN-13: 978-0-600-60993-3
ISBN-10: 0-600-60993-6

A CIP catalogue record for this book is available from the British Library

Printed and bound in China

10 9 8 7 6 5 4 3 2 1

Introduction   6
Why size matters   8
Understanding weight and fat   10
Causes of middle-age spread   12
Understanding diet basics   14
Foods to fight middle-age spread   17
Planning and motivation   20

THE WAISTLINE DIET PLAN   **22**
How the diet plan works   24
Shopping list   26
Diet maintenance plan   27

THE WAISTLINE EXERCISE PLAN   **70**
How the exercise plan works   72

Index   124
Acknowledgments   128

14 15 16 17 18 19 20 21 22 23 24 25 26

CONTENTS

INTRODUCTION

Middle-age spread is something that affects us all. It's an age-related, hormonal condition that has serious health implications. Research shows that women especially are prone to rapid weight gain in middle age, a time when hormonal changes alter metabolism and increase appetite by up to 67 percent. However, men, too, are prone to midriff spread from their thirties onward, and the health implications of the condition are no less serious for them.

THE BATTLE OF THE BULGE

The good news is that you can fight back against middle-age weight gain—and this book will show you how. The Waistline Plan is all about making small changes in the way you eat and exercise and, most importantly, in the

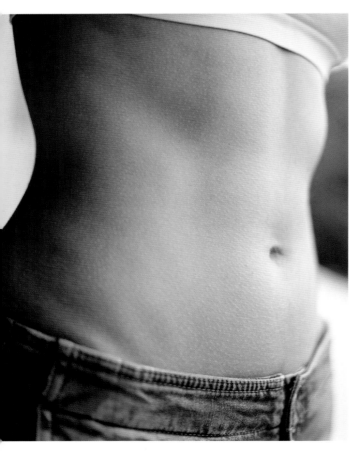

way you understand your body. Getting to know your nutritional needs, raising your metabolism, controlling your blood sugar levels, balancing your hormones, and spending a little time on exercise will help you to control the spread of excess weight around your middle, no matter what your age. By following the delicious menu plan and some simple fitness routines for just 6 weeks you can lose 14 lb; you will look and feel slimmer, fitter, and younger. Once you have achieved your target weight, you can use the Diet Maintenance Plan (see page 27) to keep the weight off for good.

The Waistline Diet Plan

The easy-to-follow 42-day menu plan includes tasty recipes, nutritional advice, ideas for healthy snacks, and tips to keep you motivated. The food options are flexible and filling, with alternatives for breakfast, lunch, and dinner, plus two nutritious snacks per day—so you won't even notice that you're on a diet and you and your family certainly won't get bored!

The Waistline Exercise Plan

You don't have to spend hours exercising to make a difference. Just 10 minutes of toning exercises, repeated 3 times a day, 5 days a week, combined with a single weekly session of aerobic exercise, will have a fantastic impact on your health and fitness. With only minor adjustments to your usual schedule, you'll be able to lose that excess weight and tone up your body. All the toning exercises are specifically designed to target the areas where middle-age spread is common—around the stomach, waist, hips, thighs, and buttocks.

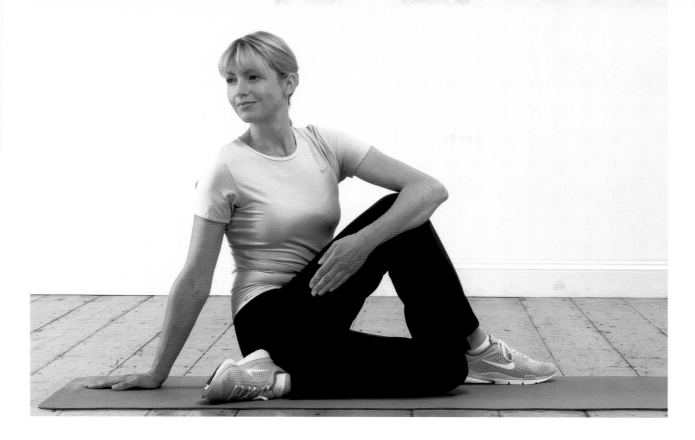

WHAT'S SPECIAL ABOUT THE PLAN?

The Waistline Plan really works, because it's not based on any faddish or very demanding regimes. It simply combats the nutritional, medical and lifestyle causes of middle-age spread with a simple approach to healthy eating and exercise that can be adopted by anyone.

- Unlike other diets, the Waistline Diet Plan doesn't deprive you of food. It actively encourages you to eat —and shows you how to make the right food choices.
- Regular, healthy meals and snacks each day will help to stabilize your blood sugar levels and eliminate those unhealthy cravings.
- The menus include foods to boost your metabolism and balance your hormones, both of which can have a huge effect in helping you to keep weight off your middle.
- You won't be cutting out any important food groups, but you will reduce your intake of sugar and salt. You do eat fats—but only those that are good for you.
- There is no need to calorie count.
- The whole family will enjoy the recipes, so there is no need to cook different meals.
- The Waistline Exercise Plan is very flexible and specially designed to fit into busy lives. Workouts can be as short as 10 minutes, but you can easily make them longer.
- Toning and aerobic exercise together produce great results, by burning fat and firming up your body.

WHY MOST DIETS DON'T WORK

Diets often fail because people get bored with them or because they limit food intake so excessively that dieters find themselves hungry and craving certain foods—and just end up reaching for those cookies or candies. There are also nutritional reasons why "yo-yo" dieters so often fail. Depriving the body of food simply places it in a fasting state, making it hang onto the fat you are trying to shift. Starvation causes the metabolism to slow down, so there is a danger of putting on weight as soon as you eat normally. What's more, when the body's intake of food is restricted it becomes stressed. Stress causes blood sugar levels to fluctuate, creating excess glucose with nowhere to go except to make more fat (see page 12).

This book will help you to understand the nutritional needs of your body. You'll find out what makes your hormones swing into action and cause weight gain, how aging changes your body and how stress can have a dangerous effect on your wellbeing. This information will enable you to manage the lifestyle changes you are about to make through the Waistline Plan.

WHY SIZE MATTERS

Middle-age spread is part of a recognized medical condition known as the somatopause. It can have serious consequences, affecting your energy, memory, mood, and libido, as well as your muscle and bone density, skin quality, and cholesterol levels, and increasing the risk of disease. You may only be in your mid-thirties, but your body will look and act older than your age. By showing you how to fight middle-age spread, the Waistline Plan will help to restore your vitality and give you the chance of leading a longer, healthier life.

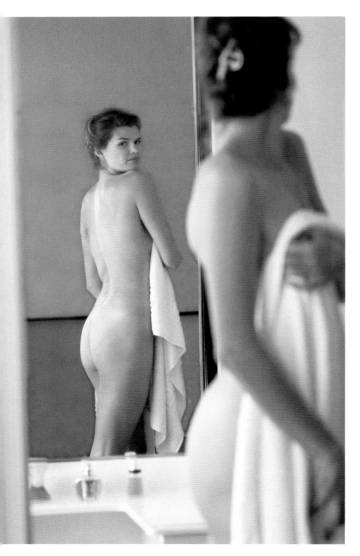

Heart disease and stroke

Heart disease is one of the biggest causes of disability and death in the West. People who eat a typical Western diet tend to accumulate fatty deposits on their artery walls, which leads to arteriosclerosis (narrowing and hardening of the arteries). This can cause angina, severe chest pain, stroke, and heart attack. Overweight people are also more likely to suffer from hypertension (raised blood pressure), increasing the risk of heart disease and stroke.

If you are overweight, reducing your weight by 10 percent can decrease your risk of developing heart disease, reduce your blood pressure, and also lower the levels of "bad" low-density lipoprotein (LDL) cholesterol and triglycerides (which are also fats) in your blood.

Diabetes

Statistically, overweight people—those with a Body Mass Index (BMI) of 25 or over (see page 10)—are twice as likely to develop Type 2 diabetes as people who are not overweight. Non insulin-dependent diabetes mellitus (Type 2 diabetes) is the most common type of diabetes in the West. It is a long-term condition, in which the body is unable to regulate the amount of glucose (sugar) in the blood properly. It occurs when the body no longer responds adequately to the natural hormone insulin (see page 12) or when the production of insulin is too low.

The good news is that Type 2 diabetes can usually be controlled through diet, exercise, and medication. If poorly controlled, it increases the risk of heart disease, strokes, nerve damage, and blindness. People who are an "apple shape"—with lots of fat around the abdomen— are at greater risk of developing this type of diabetes.

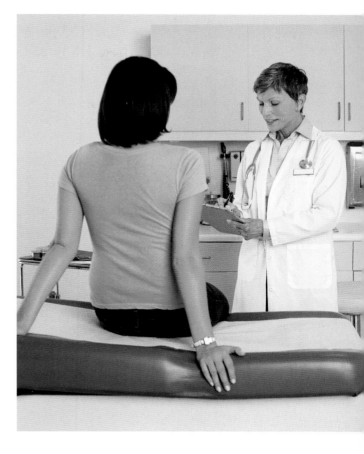

WHY EXERCISE IS GOOD FOR YOU

- Exercise increases your energy and self-confidence.
- It also controls cortisol, one of the hunger hormones (see page 12).
- Exercise helps to reduce your blood pressure, lower your heart rate and reduce your risk of stroke, heart disease, diabetes, osteoporosis, and other debilitating conditions.
- Just 10 minutes of exercise, repeated 3 times a day, 5 days a week will make a difference.

Osteoarthritis

This is a common and painful joint disorder that most often affects the joints in the knees, hips, and lower back. Being overweight appears to increase the risk of osteoarthritis, by placing extra pressure on the joints and wearing away the cartilage—the tissue that cushions the joints and normally protects them.

Cancer

Several types of cancer are associated with obesity. In women, these include cancer of the uterus, gallbladder, cervix, ovary, breast, and colon. Overweight men are at greater risk of developing cancer of the colon, rectum, and prostate.

For some types of cancer, such as colon or breast, it is not clear whether the increased risk is due to the extra weight or to a high-fat and high-calorie diet—this, of course, being strongly associated with weight problems.

Gallbladder disease

Gallbladder disease is most often caused by gallstones. These are more common in people who are overweight, and the risk of the disease increases as weight increases. It is thought that the condition is caused by changes in the way the body handles fat and cholesterol, leading to an over-saturation of bile.

Sleep apnea

This is a serious condition that is closely associated with being overweight. It can cause a person to stop breathing for short periods during sleep and to snore heavily. As a further consequence, there may be daytime sleepiness and, in extreme cases, the onset of symptoms of heart failure. The risk of sleep apnea increases with higher body weights.

Fatigue

Being overweight makes you tired, not just because of the extra weight you are carrying but also due to changes in hormone production as the body gradually becomes insulin resistant (see pages 12–13). As a consequence, you will become increasingly tired, and in the long run you may develop Type 2 diabetes.

Back pain

Any excess weight places extra strain on your body, and if you are carrying excess weight around your middle then it is more than likely that your stomach muscles are not being exercised and are weak. Strong stomach muscles support the back and help prevent back pain.

Infertility

Being overweight reduces a woman's chances of becoming pregnant, as it affects hormone production and ovulation.

UNDERSTANDING WEIGHT AND FAT

Two methods can be used to identify whether you are overweight. Body Mass Index (BMI) is used internationally as a way of determining whether your weight is putting your health at risk. BMI considers weight and height and it is best used in conjunction with the waist-to-hip ratio (WHR) measurement, which calculates your percentage of body fat. Some professionals consider your WHR to be more accurate for assessing health risks, as it measures abdominal fat—the fat most associated with health problems.

BODY MASS INDEX

There are two ways of finding out if you are the right weight for your height. Refer to the weight-height chart (right) to see if you are underweight, normal weight, overweight, obese, or severely obese. If your weight is at the lower end of the normal range, try to maintain it and don't be tempted to aim for the underweight category.

Calculating your BMI

You can also use this method to calculate your BMI:

1 Measure your height in meters and multiply this figure by itself.
2 Measure your weight in kilograms.
3 Divide the weight by height squared. For example, the BMI for someone who weighs 10 stone (140 lb/65 kg) and is 5 ft 7 in (1.7 m) tall is: 65 divided by (1.7 x 1.7) = 22.5. This weight would be within the normal range.

What does it mean?

below 18.5	underweight
18.5–25	normal weight
25–30	overweight
30–35	obese
above 35	severely obese

The range from 18.5 to 25 is quite wide, as "normal" weight-for-height covers men and women and people of different shapes and body composition. A man usually has a higher BMI than a woman of the same height, as men tend to have more muscle (muscle weighs more than fat). A slim, muscular woman will have a higher BMI than a slim, not very muscular woman of the same height.

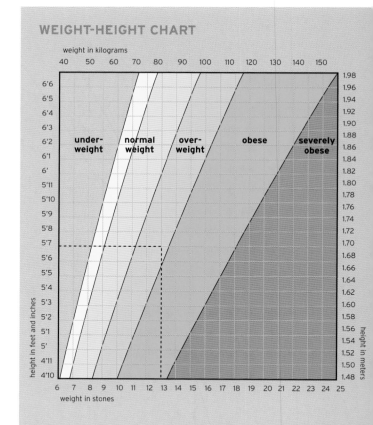

WEIGHT-HEIGHT CHART

The example shown by the dotted line describes the BMI of someone who is 5 ft 7 in (1.7 m) tall and weighs 13 stone (182 lb/82 kg). This gives a BMI in the top end of the overweight category.

WAIST-TO-HIP RATIO

The waist-to-hip ratio (WHR) is used to determine how much body fat you are carrying. This measurement is thought to be a more reliable guide to your risk of health problems than the BMI calculation, as it is possible to have a high BMI and a normal waist measurement if, for example, you are a fit, lean, muscular man.

You can work out your WHR by dividing your waist measurement by your hip measurement. For women, the ratio should not be over 0.85; for men, it should not be over 0.90. The higher the number above these values, the greater the risk of heart disease and other problems.

Calculating your WHR

1 Measure your waist circumference at the narrowest part. Slowly breathe out—don't hold in your stomach. Do not pull the tape too tight.
2 Measure your hip circumference at the widest part.
3 Divide your waist measurement by your hip measurement. For example, the WHR of a woman with a waist measuring 35 in and hips measuring 41 in is: 35 divided by 41 = 0.85. This measurement is at the top end of the normal range.

WAIST CIRCUMFERENCE

In addition to the BMI and WHR calculations, you can use your waist circumference measurement to evaluate whether you are at risk of obesity complications and mortality. In women, a waist circumference above 35 in confers increased risk. In men, the risks begin to rise at a measurement of 40 in.

ALL ABOUT BODY FAT

Normal levels of fat are not a problem for the body. Fat is an energy reservoir, laid down when food is plentiful and converted back to energy when needed. However, when too much of the wrong kind of food is consumed, and calorie intake is higher than calorie expenditure, weight is accumulated. Eventually, this can lead to obesity.

Fat may be subcutaneous or visceral. Subcutaneous fat lies just under the skin, while visceral fat is stored deep inside the body. It is the visceral fat in the midriff section of the body (sometimes known as intra-abdominal fat) and its proximity to the portal vein—a major vessel that feeds the liver—that increase the risk of disease. Visceral fat releases substances that may flow directly into the liver and set off a chain of events that can lead to insulin resistance and the suppression of leptin, a hormone-like substance that tells the brain when you are full (see pages 12–13).

Most fat is stored under the skin, but, as well as visceral fat, there is also some on top of the kidneys and inside the liver and muscles. Other body parts that gather fat depend on gender: men are prone to storing fat on the chest, middle, and buttocks (apple shape), while women accumulate fat on the breasts, waist, hips, buttocks, and thighs (pear shape). Following the drop in estrogen levels after the menopause, women too begin to accumulate fat around the middle.

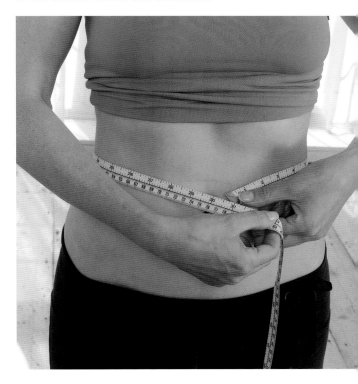

CAUSES OF MIDDLE-AGE SPREAD

While genetics play a role in the accumulation of middle-age spread, it doesn't have to be a fact of life. From lack of exercise and unbalanced hormones to stress and pollutants, there are many reasons why you may gain weight around your abdomen and hips as you get older. The Waistline Plan tackles middle-age spread by addressing its underlying causes, whether through exercise or by foods that balance hormones and boost the metabolism (see pages 17–19).

Hormones

The hormones directly related to appetite include leptin, insulin, and ghrelin. When working in harmony they help to maintain a healthy body weight, but factors including stress, lifestyle, and processed foods can knock them off balance and result in weight gain. A healthy diet that includes foods which help to balance your hormones can help you to lose weight (see pages 17–18).

- **Leptin** This hormone suppresses appetite. Produced by fatty tissues, it travels to the hypothalamus, the brain's appetite center, where it induces satiation. At the same time, it stimulates the nervous system, urging the body to increase its metabolism. When leptin levels in the blood and brain drop, the signal to eat takes over again.

- **Ghrelin** This recently discovered hunger hormone both stimulates the desire to eat and controls the feeling of hunger. The levels of ghrelin fall when you eat, but this is affected by the type of food: carbohydrates have the greatest effect and fat the smallest. You are much more likely to feel hungrier, quicker, after eating fatty food than a carbohydrate-rich meal.

- **Insulin** Produced by the pancreas, this hormone regulates carbohydrate metabolism. Secretion of insulin increases rapidly after eating. Most body cells have insulin receptors that bind circulating insulin, allowing glucose (sugar) to be absorbed from the bloodstream into cells. However, when you are overweight, high levels of uncontrolled insulin circulate within your body. Excess insulin may also be released if blood sugar increases constantly as a reaction to stress (see below). If the glucose is not used up it is stored as fat and, furthermore, the continual production of insulin eventually makes the body insulin resistant. It will then be difficult for you to lose weight, and you will also increase your chances of developing Type 2 diabetes (see page 8).

Stress

One of the biggest contributors to increasing abdominal fat, stress affects the adrenal glands. These are located near the kidneys and produce the hormones cortisol and adrenalin, releasing them into the bloodstream. When healthy, the adrenals increase heart rate and blood pressure, release energy stores for immediate use, slow digestion, and sharpen the senses. Under continual stress, however, they remain on constant alert.

DID YOU KNOW?

- Natural sunlight is an appetite suppressant, as it helps to regulate hormones associated with hunger. You typically eat less when the weather is warm and sunny.

- During the perimenopause and menopause, erratic hormone fluctuations can cause rapid weight gain and changes in body shape.

- Women's bodies are more prone to hormonal imbalance than men's. Women gain weight, lose weight and maintain weight at certain times of their lives due to physiological, psychological, cultural, or emotional factors.

Levels of adrenalin fall as soon as the stress subsides, but cortisol remains in the body much longer. This hormone sends a message to the brain to refuel, believing the body has used up large amounts of energy. As a consequence, you will eat more food than is actually necessary and put on weight. The deep fat cells in the belly are especially good at attracting cortisol, which causes them to release fat into the bloodstream and the excess to be stored as a layer of fat below the abdominal muscle. At the same time, the foods you often crave when you are stressed—cookies, chocolate, cakes —raise blood sugar and therefore levels of insulin. High levels of sugar and insulin encourage your body to store fat and lead to insulin resistance.

Aging and menopause

From around the age of 30, muscle mass gradually decreases each year and, as muscle is metabolically very active, causes a decline in the body's overall metabolic rate. There is also a decline in the growth hormone as you age, which is thought to contribute to weight gain around the middle. Most women find that their weight starts to increase particularly around the perimenopause, the years leading up to the menopause. This is because fat helps in the production of estrogen, which reduces during menopause. The body will attempt to keep estrogen levels high by holding onto the fat.

Exercise and metabolism

Your metabolism slows down as you age and you need to boost it through exercise. Building muscles through strength training is also very important, as muscles are metabolically active and continue to burn calories even at rest. Between the ages of 40 and 50 you will lose around 1 lb of muscle per year, and women lose muscle mass faster than men. Physical activity also helps to control the production of stress hormones (see above).

Body fat percentage

Fat is less metabolically active than muscle, meaning it requires fewer calories to sustain it. This is why body fat percentage is so important for weight control: the higher your percentage of fat (and the smaller your percentage of muscle), the fewer calories you need to maintain your weight and therefore the easier it is to gain weight.

Sleep

Lack of sleep can also adversely affect appetite as levels of leptin drop and ghrelin rise. Serotonin is another hormone affected by sleep and stress, and is also a contributing factor in controlling your appetite.

Serotonin produces the "feel good" factor. When levels of this hormone are low, depression and apathy are likely to set in alongside weight gain—the lower your serotonin, the more you eat. Low serotonin levels can lead to food cravings (particularly for refined carbohydrates), low energy levels, and compulsive eating. Women naturally have less serotonin in their brains than men.

Pollutants

Every day your body is subjected to environmental pollutants. Found in the atmosphere you breathe, in food packaging, or sprayed onto and added to your food, these agrichemical residues and food additives are stored within your fat cells, disrupting your body's natural hormonal balance.

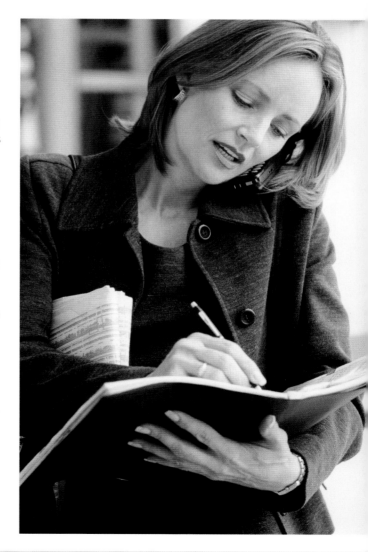

UNDERSTANDING DIET BASICS

To diet successfully you need to know the basic nutritional requirements of your body: a balance of carbohydrates, protein, healthy fats, fiber, minerals, and vitamins, consumed in moderation. It is also helpful to understand the importance of keeping blood sugar levels steady and controlling portion size, as well as the counter-productive effects of calorie counting. The Waistline Diet Plan takes all these factors into consideration, offering nourishing menus that keep you feeling full even as you lose weight.

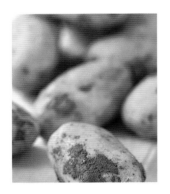
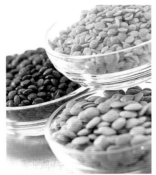
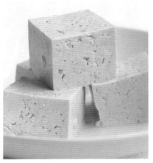
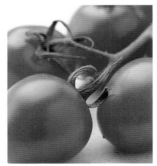
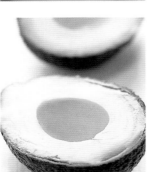
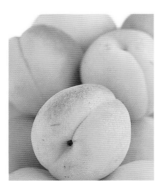

Carbohydrates

Carbohydrates give you energy to breathe, grow, move, function, and repair. There are two types of carbohydrate: simple and complex. Simple carbohydrates provide sugar, some in a natural form as found in fruit and vegetables, others in refined form in foods such as cakes, cookies and fruit concentrates. Complex carbohydrates are starch based and are found in foods such as bread, cereals, pasta, rice, millet, and legumes. Complex carbohydrates are healthier than simple carbohydrates.

Protein

Protein is required for growth and strength, as well as for muscle regeneration and hormone production. Protein is found in meat, poultry, eggs, and fish, as well as in the vegetarian alternatives of tofu, nuts, seeds, and legumes. It is also found in bread, rice, and pasta.

Fiber

Fiber is necessary for the disposal of waste from the body. Particularly good sources are wholegrain bread and cereals, brown rice, vegetables, fruit, nuts, and legumes.

Vitamins and minerals

Vitamins and minerals are vital for your body's everyday functioning. A balanced diet that includes wholegrains, fruit and vegetables, and fish, meat, or legumes should provide you with your daily requirements. Choosing organic fruit and vegetables will help you to avoid the risk of residual pesticides. At certain times, such as during the menopause, you may consider taking a vitamin and mineral supplement.

Fats

Weight-for-weight, fat provides twice as many calories as carbohydrates or protein. If you eat too much, it is stored as adipose tissue (fat around the middle). Polyunsaturated and monounsaturated fats have the same calorie content as saturated fats, but are better for your health.

- **Saturated fat** This sort of fat is largely responsible for obesity, raised levels of "bad" LDL cholesterol, hardening of the arteries, heart disease, some cancers, and strokes. It also stimulates over-production of estrogen, which can result in premenstrual and hormonal problems. Cutting down will help you to lose weight and keep you healthier. Saturated fat should be eaten only in moderation in foods such as eggs, broiled bacon, lamb, beef, and hard cheese.
- **Polyunsaturated fat** This fat supplies the body with vitamins A, D, and E, helps your hormones to stay in balance, supports your immune system, stimulates the metabolism, improves mood and brain function, and keeps cell membranes healthy and joints supple. It is found in liquid fats and oils, including vegetable oil, corn oil, and sunflower oil (palm oil should be avoided). It contains the essential fatty acids (EFAs) omega-3 and omega-6. You need to consume a variety of EFAs.

- **Omega-6** (linoleic fatty acid) is found mainly in oils including hemp, walnut, soybean, and wheatgerm, and in seeds such as pumpkin and sesame.
- **Omega-3** (alpha linoleic fatty acid) is found in oily fish like salmon, herring, tuna, sardines, and mackerel, oils such as canola, soybean, and linseed (an especially good source), nuts and seeds, green leafy vegetables, wholegrains, and spirulina (seaweed).
- **Monounsaturated fat**, also known as omega-9, is also found in liquid form, but can solidify when cooled. It offers the benefits of polyunsaturated fat and also lowers levels of "bad" LDL cholesterol and raises levels of "good" high-density lipoprotein (HDL) cholesterol. It is linked to lower rates of heart disease and some cancers. Olive oil is the best source of this fat, along with canola and sesame seed oils, avocados, and olives themselves.
- **Trans fats** are "good" vegetable fats that have been altered by food processing to improve their shelf life, texture, and flavor. Often labeled as hydrogenated fats or hydrogenated vegetable oil, they are found in cakes, cookies, pies, pastries, margarines, and take outs. They are as harmful as saturated fats to health, so try to cut them out altogether.

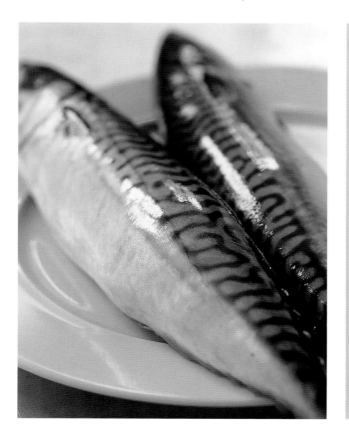

FAT-REDUCTION STRATEGIES

No more than 30 percent of your total daily calorie intake should come from fat sources. 1 g of fat provides 9 calories, so, in a diet of 1500 calories per day, your total fat intake should not exceed 2 oz (50 g), with no more than 10 percent of this being saturated fat. Here are some tips for reducing fat intake:

- Replace whole milk with skim, lowfat, or soy milk.
- Use butter and spreads sparingly.
- If using mayonnaise on bread, don't add butter or another spread as well.
- Steam, broil, or poach foods, rather than frying.
- Avoid take-out foods.
- Cut off the surplus fat from meat.
- Remove the skin from poultry.
- Limit your consumption of hard and full-fat cheeses.

COUNTING CALORIES

We all know that to lose weight you need to eat fewer calories, and use up the calories you do eat (this is especially true as you get older and your metabolism slows down). To lose weight sensibly, women should consume around 1,500 calories per day and men 2,000 calories per day. The average to maintain weight is 2,000 calories per day for women and 2,500 for men. However, all too often diets that offer a quick weight loss by cutting calories drastically can be difficult to maintain and leave you feeling deprived, depressed, and miserable.

Low-calorie foods often adversely affect your blood sugar levels. For example, a breakfast of coffee, skim milk and low-calorie cereal may be a slimming meal, but the foods themselves are simple carbohydrates, lacking in fiber and protein. Once eaten they will be broken down quickly, blood sugar will rise dramatically and then fall just as quickly, leaving you feeling hungry around mid-morning and likely to snack. Many processed "diet" foods are also full of chemicals and preservatives. The menus in the Waistline Diet Plan are built around wholesome, fresh foods that are high in nutritional value and won't leave you feeling empty.

GLYCEMIC INDEX

When you eat, the food is converted into glucose that your body uses for energy. It is the hormone insulin that controls levels of glucose, storing it when there is too much in the body and releasing it when there is too little. If glucose levels are too high, high levels of insulin (see page 12) are released and the excess glucose is quickly

stored away as fat. If you eat foods that raise glucose levels too high, you will produce too much insulin, increase your fat stores, and gain weight. You may also develop insulin resistance. Conversely, if you choose foods that are slow to raise glucose levels this will help to keep insulin production under control.

The glycemic index (GI) tells you how quickly a food raises blood sugar levels. Foods that are converted more slowly into glucose have a low GI value, while those causing a rapid and massive rise in blood sugar have a high GI value. Foods that break down quickly in the body —such as white bread, white rice, and sugary treats— have the highest GI, while foods that take longer to be digested—such as new potatoes, whole-wheat pasta, and multigrain bread—have a lower GI.

The theory behind diets based on the glycemic index is that foods with a low GI value release sugar slowly into the blood, providing you with a steady supply of energy that keeps you feeling satisfied for longer, so that you're less likely to snack. In contrast, foods with a high GI value cause a rapid but short-lived rise in blood sugar levels. This leaves you lacking in energy and feeling hungry again within a short time, so that you end up reaching for another carbohydrate "fix." It is these highs and lows that result in hunger and excess weight gain.

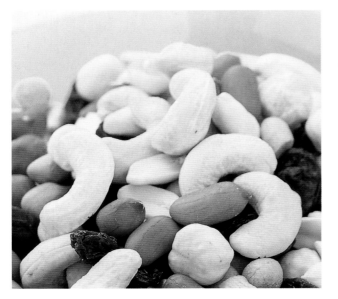

FOODS TO FIGHT
MIDDLE-AGE SPREAD

Some foods are especially beneficial in combating middle-age weight gain and promoting good health and wellbeing. The menus in the Waistline Diet Plan are built around foods that will help to control the hormones, such as cortisol and insulin, that are associated with weight gain. The ingredients used in the meals will also help to reduce the effects of stress and pollution, and they will boost your metabolism, increasing the rate at which you burn off calories.

REGULATING HORMONES

The body's endocrine system is responsible for releasing chemical messengers—your hormones—into the bloodstream. Unfortunately, hormones can be disrupted easily. Gaining weight, particularly around your middle, is linked to stress-related disruption of cortisol, which is secreted from the adrenal glands. Another factor in weight gain is overproduction of insulin, caused by an excess of blood sugar. (See pages 12–13 for more on the role of hormones.) Synthetic chemicals found in agrichemicals, food additives and preservatives, plastic packaging, and so on also disrupt the body's endocrine system, by mimicking natural hormones.

Foods to balance hormones

A healthy diet helps to balance the endocrine system. Broccoli, for example, is a great source of chromium, a trace mineral that helps the pancreas to function properly and therefore increases insulin efficiency, which in turn helps to regulate blood sugar levels. Other foods you should include in your diet are:

- **Complex carbohydrates** Wholegrains, bread, rice, legumes, leafy green vegetables.
- **Vitamin B3** Yeast extract, wheat bran, turkey, chicken, fish, wholegrains, mushrooms, milk products.
- **Vitamin B6** Meat and dairy products, bananas, broccoli, red kidney beans, cauliflower, cabbage, watercress.
- **Zinc** Beef, lamb, calf's liver, turkey, sardines, crab, oyster, Brazil nuts, eggs, pumpkin seeds, yeast.
- **Protein** Chicken, meat, fish, eggs, milk, tofu, soya, quinoa.
- **Essential fatty acids (EFAs)** Oily fish, olive oil, nuts and seeds.

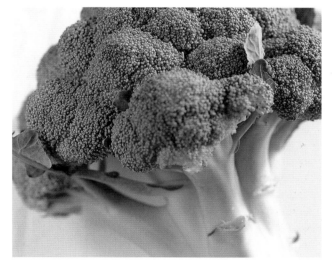

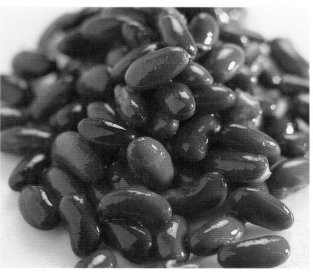

Foods to control insulin production

When you eat carbohydrates, your body responds by producing the hormone insulin. Good carbohydrates (see pages 14–16) are the key to keeping insulin production under control and the weight off. They are found in brown and basmati rice, oats, rye, millet, legumes, cherries, apples, pears, grapefruit, oranges, plums, dried apricots, green vegetables (leafy green ones, as well as zucchini, squashes, green sweet peppers, cucumber, artichokes, celery), onions, garlic, and tomatoes.

Foods to control stress hormones

Stress affects your adrenal glands by changing the behavior of adrenal hormones (see pages 12–13). These hormones are responsible for many symptoms of stress, such as high blood pressure, digestive upset, muscle tension, and, of course, fat around the middle. If the stress continues for a period of time, the adrenal glands can become exhausted. Foods high in nutrients that support adrenal gland function include:

- **Celery** Helps you to sleep if eaten at night; also helps to lower blood pressure.
- **Brown rice** Complex carbohydrate that helps to release serotonin, the feel-good, calming chemical that lifts mood and boosts energy.
- **Cabbage** Full of the antioxidant vitamins A, C, and E, beta-carotene, and the mineral selenium. Also releases serotonin for mood-boosting effects.
- **Sunflower seeds** Rich in vitamin B, zinc, and potassium, all of which are heavily depleted by stress.
- **Berries** Rich in manganese and vitamin C to boost the immune system.

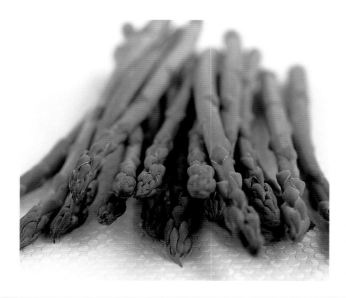

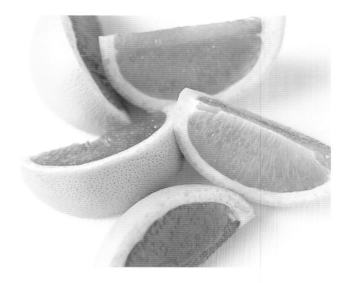

- **Avocados** Packed with beneficial polyunsaturated fats and minerals that stimulate the growth hormone and boost the metabolism.
- **Asparagus** Rich in the enzymes that help to regulate mood swings.
- **Sesame seeds** Source of zinc and useful in the metabolism of fatty acids and serotonin.

FIGHTING POLLUTION

Anitoxidants include vitamins A, C, and E, selenium, carotenoids, and phytochemicals. These substances protect your body against the damaging effects of an excess of "free radicals," sources of which include pollution, sunlight, tobacco fumes, radiation, stress, and illness. Excess free radicals cause cell damage and this is thought to lead to an increased risk of cancer, heart disease, and arthritis. Antioxidants in your diet help to neutralize the free radicals in your body and halt their damaging effects.

- **Fruit and vegetables** Eat a wide variety—including sweet potatoes, carrots, spinach, and mangoes—to provide you with plenty of antioxidants.
- **Green tea** This helps to protect your organs and flushes out toxins and pollutants.
- **Milk thistle** Use a supplement to protect your liver from toxins.

THE ROLE OF METABOLISM

Your metabolism is the rate at which your body burns calories in order to keep itself alive and it is always working, even when you are sleeping. Encouraging your metabolism to work more effectively is therefore a key factor in losing weight.

After the age of 30, your metabolic rate begins to drop by around 1 percent each year, and as a result older dieters often complain that they cannot lose weight. But your metabolism can be boosted—you just need to know how and when.

How to boost metabolism

Your metabolism has 3 different aspects: the basal or resting metabolism; the activity metabolism; and the thermic or digestive metabolism. To boost your metabolism efficiently, you need to raise all 3 metabolic rates. To do this you need to:

- Eat first thing in the morning to kick-start your metabolism, and eat regularly throughout the day to prevent peaks and troughs in insulin production and carbohydrate metabolism (see pages 12–13).
- Exercise to build muscle and stimulate the growth hormone, as this helps to raise your basal metabolism. Any exercise also boosts your activity metabolism.
- Eat foods that contain protein, fiber, calcium, and spices to boost your thermic and basal metabolisms.

Foods to boost metabolism

Certain foods take more energy to digest them, so it is worth including these in your diet to help to speed up your metabolism:

- **Complex carbohydrates** release energy slowly and boost your metabolism by keeping insulin levels low after you eat.
- **Calcium** Milk is one of the best foods for providing calcium, which boosts your basal metabolism. Other dairy products and leafy green vegetables are also good sources.
- **Protein** Protein is harder to digest than other food groups, so more energy is used by the body to break it down and therefore more calories are consumed.
- **Omega-3 oils** These alter the levels of leptin in the body, a hormone directly related to metabolism and responsible for whether you burn or store fat (see page 12). Low levels of leptin mean you burn more fat, and omega-3 reduces leptin levels. If you really don't like fish, or are vegetarian, then you can take an essential fatty acid supplement.
- **Fiber** Foods high in fiber boost your metabolism, as they take longer to digest.
- **Capsaicin** Found in sweet peppers, this really raises your metabolism as it speeds up your heart rate. Peppers make a great snack option and the effect of capsaicin persists for several hours after you have

DID YOU KNOW?

- Between 60 and 80 percent of your daily calories are burned up doing nothing! This is because even when you are asleep (or just resting) your heart is beating, your organs are functioning, and your lungs are breathing. Only around 30 percent of the calories you consume each day are used up during activity.
- Every day, the average woman burns about 10 calories for every 1 lb of body weight; the average man burns 11 calories.

finished eating. It is also found in chili spices, which you can add to your food.

- **Chromium** This trace mineral works with insulin to metabolize fats and carbohydrates, and a deficiency can cause blood sugar to soar and fat/carbohydrate metabolism to drop radically. Adding a chromium supplement to your diet will help to stabilize your blood sugar levels.
- **Water** Dehydration slows your thermic metabolism—you need water in your stomach in order to digest food. Aim to drink 8 glasses or 10 cups of fluid per day. Drinking enough water may be hard, but fruit juice can be a source as well as herbal tea.
- **Green tea** This type of tea contains a phytochemical known as ECGC, which researchers believe can boost your basal metabolism.

PLANNING AND MOTIVATION

You may have bought this book because you have a special party or vacation coming up and you want to look great in that new dress or bikini. Or maybe your health is suffering and you realize it is time to take stock, or perhaps you feel down and depressed. Whatever your reasons for starting the Waistline Plan, you will find that following it brings a whole range of different benefits, including increased energy, a positive frame of mind, and a guilt-free attitude to food—not to mention a new waistline!

MAKE THAT COMMITMENT

For the initial 6 weeks of the Waistline Plan, make a commitment to your body and your health and fitness. Look at the Waistline Plan as being the most important thing in your life for the next 6 weeks: if you are totally committed to it, you will be surprised at how easily others accept your plans.

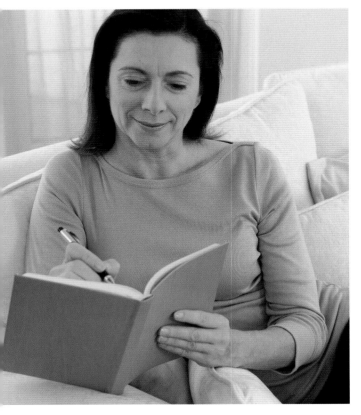

Set attainable goals, write them down and leave them in a place where you can see them every day, like on the door of the refrigerator or next to the phone. It's a good idea to set both short- and long-term goals, so you can cross off the short-term ones as you achieve them. Simple goals, such as not eating chocolate for 4 days or exercising for 10 minutes every day, may not sound much to others, but they will have a positive effect and make you realize just what you can achieve.

GOOD PLANNING

Planning ahead at every stage is the key to motivation and will help you to overcome any obstacles. Set a day to start, but preferably not a Monday—halfway through the week is much better psychologically. Avoid booking in any heavy social engagements or vacations during the first few weeks, which would impose extra pressure on you, and don't accept offers that may sabotage your efforts, such as an outing to a restaurant.

Empty your refrigerator and kitchen cabinets of all the food that is simply no good for you. Out go all processed foods such as white bread, cookies, cakes, chips, candy, crackers, white pasta, white rice, and sauces, along with ready meals and anything that isn't fresh and fruity. Stock up on the items listed on the shopping list (see page 26) before you start the plan, buying fresh fruit, vegetables, meat, and fish as required during the course of the plan.

If you intend to swap days and meals around, plan this out on a weekly schedule and pin it up where you can see it easily. Include your snacks in the list and have them readily to hand or if necessary make them up, especially if you will be out and about for the day.

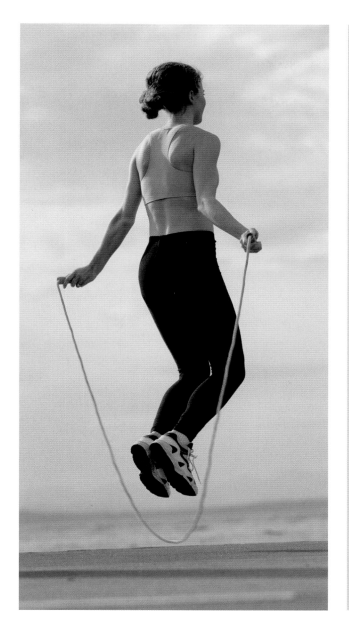

Like any new regime, there may be times when you find the Waistline Plan challenging. Here are some tips for keeping going:

- Make a list of all the reasons you are doing the Waistline Plan and put it somewhere where you will see it every day.
- Build in some rewards: celebrate the completion of the first week with a massage, manicure, or trip to the movies.
- Boost your metabolism by climbing stairs, skipping, and walking that extra mile. The fitter you become, the easier it will be to follow the Waistline Plan.
- Exercising with a friend or partner will increase your commitment and make you work harder.
- Buy some attractive new workout wear to make exercise even more enjoyable.
- Think positively about exercise. If you experience a negative thought, push it away with a positive affirmation such as "This will reduce my waistline."
- Vary your workouts to keep them fresh.
- Chart your success, keeping a record of what you have eaten, how many times you have exercised, and how much weight you have lost. Measure your chest, waist, hips, and each thigh before you begin the plan, every other week during the plan, and again when you have completed it.

Whenever you start to get low on ingredients, make another shopping list and stick to it. If necessary, try internet shopping so that you won't be tempted by other foods when you get into the store.

Plan your toning and aerobic workouts for the week, then write them down in a simple chart form and pin this up beside your menu plan. Make sure you specify the times when you intend to work out on the chart and on your calendar—make a promise to yourself that you won't miss any of them. The best time to exercise is in the morning, as this will boost your metabolism for the rest of the day. Remember: you can fit in that extra 10 minutes if you want to! It's a good idea to stick to the same times each day to exercise. If you get into a regular routine it will be easier to maintain.

You can always set yourself some personal exercise targets, such as adding another 10-minute exercise session into each day for the last week. Plan how you will treat yourself if you meet your targets; this will encourage you and help you to recognize your success.

If you really can't find time to exercise, perhaps because of unusually heavy work commitments, then at least try to walk further that day. Park the car away from the office, walk to the stores or in the park at lunchtime. Walk briskly to maximize the benefits. There are always ways to exercise a little more!

THE WAISTLINE

| 1 | 2 | 3 | 4 | 5 | 6 | 7 | 8 | 9 | 10 | 11 | 12 | 13 |

DIET PLAN

14 15 16 17 18 19 20 21 22 23 24 25 26

HOW THE DIET PLAN WORKS

The Waistline Diet Plan is not, in fact, a restrictive "diet," but a positive change in your eating habits. You don't have to count calories all the time—just eat sensibly from a range of menu options, following the guidelines about portion size and ingredients. Feeding and nourishing your body properly, combined with taking more exercise, will help to boost your metabolism, stabilize blood sugar levels, and regulate hormones. This is the only successful way of losing that excess weight around your middle.

WHAT DOES THE PLAN OFFER?

The Waistline Diet Plan sets out the next 42 days for you. Decide when you want to start, plan ahead using the shopping list on page 26, then follow the daily menus. These will provide the nutritious and balanced diet you need to lose that excess weight around your middle.

For convenience, you can occasionally mix and match meals on different days. For example, you may want to replace dinner on day 3 with dinner on day 10, or lunch on day 7 with lunch on day 12—but do not replace a lunch with an extra dinner, or vice versa.

Nourishing your body

When you embark on the Waistline Diet Plan, you should eat a breakfast, lunch, and dinner option and the snacks from each day's menu. Note that the dessert course applies to both main course alternatives, unless two desserts have been specified (in that case go with the dessert option that accompanies your chosen main course). The menus provide the right quantities of carbohydrate, protein, fats, vitamins, minerals, and fiber for your daily needs. They also contain the ingredients that fight the causes of middle-age spread (see pages 12–13). You will be eating foods that balance hormones, control insulin production, counteract the effects of stress and pollution, and boost your metabolism.

Meal schedule

When following the Waistline Diet Plan, you will be eating little and often. This will help to stabilize your blood sugar levels and prevent cravings for carbohydrates and sweet things. Ideally, you should try to eat your dinner before

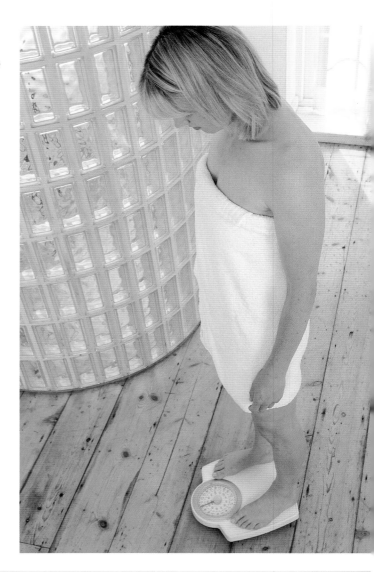

7.30 pm. This will allow your body time to digest your meal before going to bed, helping you to sleep better.

The Waistline Diet Plan includes two healthy snacks each day. If you get really hungry, choose another snack or a fruit smoothie (these are really filling) from the plan.

Fruit and vegetables

Suggestions are given in the menus for the types of fruit, vegetables, nuts, and seeds you can eat as snacks or to accompany a meal. This is simply to give you ideas that you might not otherwise have considered, but you can always create your own list (see the good foods discussed on pages 14–19). If possible, buy organic, fresh foods because these are the healthiest—food that is covered in pesticides and herbicides and full of additives can upset your hormonal balance and immune system.

Do not eat more than 5 pieces of fruit a day. Fruit contains its own sugar and this can ultimately affect your blood sugar levels.

Making life easy

As well as buying in the healthy ingredients you'll be using, it really is a good idea to get rid of all the foods you won't be eating. Having cookies, cakes, and pastries loitering in your pantry will make temptation much harder to resist.

If you are catering for a family, you need to prepare them too, so that they can help to support you. The Waistline Diet Plan is not just healthy, it's designed to fit into your lifestyle and it's suitable for all the family. There are lots of vegetarian options, so you should find that there's something to please everyone.

GETTING THE MOST FROM THE PLAN

- Start the day with a drink of hot water and lemon to stimulate your liver and clean out toxins from your body.

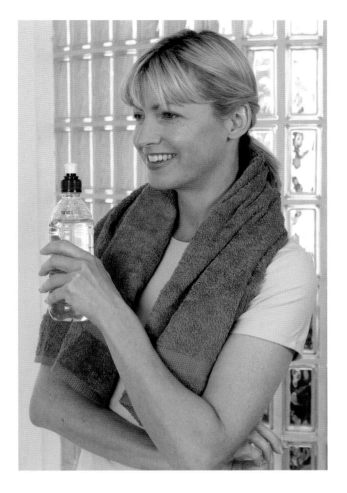

- Always eat breakfast to kick-start your metabolism for the day.
- Try to build exercise session(s) into your morning schedule, as this will raise your metabolic rate and helps to burn fat throughout the day.
- Avoid coffee and alcohol. Cut back on your tea intake, too—try herbal teas instead.
- Turn off the television, put down the newspaper and don't look at the computer screen when you eat. It is very important to register what you are eating.
- Plan ahead: make sure you have all the foods for your menu in your pantry and refrigerator.
- Do not weigh yourself daily: once a week is plenty. Remember always to weigh yourself at the same time of day.
- Treat yourself every now and then. If you have been sticking to the plan for several weeks, then allow yourself a treat – but in moderation.
- Never eat late at night—it's not good for your digestion and may interrupt your sleep.
- Get enough sleep—it helps you to burn fat.

STAY HYDRATED

Remember that you can often mistake dehydration for hunger. Drink 6–8 glasses (8–10 cups) of water per day. Your body is 70 percent fluid, a proportion of which is lost through sweat, urine, and breathing each day, so you need to replace it by drinking at regular intervals. Drink more water before, during and after exercise as well.

SHOPPING LIST

Before you begin the Waistline Diet Plan it is important to prepare yourself properly. Each day is planned, so that you know what you'll be eating and when. If you have the right ingredients to hand, there is much less chance of you snacking on something unsuitable. Below is a list of the basic foods that you'll require to follow the Waistline Diet Plan. Buy them in advance and replace them as necessary. Fresh fruit, vegetables, meat, and fish are best bought as needed during the plan and used within a few days.

CEREALS
- Cereal (crunchy oat, wholegrain breakfast)
- Granola (sugar-free)
- Oats (jumbo, rolled)

GRAINS
- Bagels
- Bread (multigrain, rye, wholegrain)
- Bulgar wheat
- Couscous
- Malt loaf
- Millet
- Noodles (buckwheat, thread egg)
- Pasta (egg, whole-wheat)
- Pearl barley
- Pitas (whole-wheat)
- Quinoa
- Rice (brown, wild)
- Rice pancakes

LEGUMES
- Beans (flageolet, kidney, lima, pinto)
- Lentils (Puy, red)
- Peas (chickpeas, split yellow peas)
- Tofu

NUTS
- Almonds
- Brazil nuts
- Cashew nuts
- Hazelnuts
- Pine nuts
- Walnuts

SEEDS
- Flax
- Pumpkin
- Sesame
- Sunflower

DRIED FRUIT
- Apricots
- Dates
- Golden raisins
- Prunes
- Raisins

DAIRY PRODUCTS
- Butter
- Cheese (cheddar, cottage cheese, lowfat cream cheese, feta, lowfat goat, mozzarella, Parmesan, ricotta)
- Eggs
- Sour cream, lowfat
- Yogurt (lowfat, plain, fruit)

DRINKS
- Fruit juices (apple, apple and mango, grapefruit, orange, pineapple, pomegranate, tomato)
- Milk (lowfat or skim)
- Soy milk
- Tea (green, herbal)
- Water (filtered, mineral)

COOKING ALCOHOL
- Calvados
- Vodka
- White wine

OILS
- Canola
- Chili-infused
- Groundnut
- Olive
- Sesame
- Sunflower

GENERAL STORES
- Almond extract
- Artichoke hearts, canned
- Berry fruits, frozen
- Capers
- Chocolate, dark
- Cream of tartar
- Flour (buckwheat, whole-wheat)
- Honey
- Hummus
- Mayonnaise, low-calorie
- Mirin
- Miso
- Mustard
- Oatcakes
- Olive oil spread
- Olives
- Orange-blossom water
- Peas, frozen
- Peanut butter
- Plum sauce
- Rice cakes
- Soy sauce
- Stock (chicken, fish, vegetable)
- Sugar (light brown, light cane, superfine)
- Sun-dried tomatoes
- Tabasco sauce
- Tahini
- Thai fish sauce
- Tomato paste
- Tomatoes, canned
- Tuna, canned
- Vegetable soup, canned
- Vinegar (balsamic, cider, rice wine, white wine)
- Wasabi
- Water chestnuts, canned

SPICES
- Allspice berries
- Black mustard seeds
- Black peppercorns
- Cardamom
- Cayenne pepper
- Chili powder
- Cinnamon
- Cloves
- Coriander seeds
- Cumin seeds
- Fennel seeds
- Garam masala
- Ground coriander
- Ground cumin
- Ground mace
- Ground turmeric
- Lemon pepper
- Nutmeg
- Onion seeds
- Paprika
- Rock salt
- Saffron threads
- Star anise

FOODS TO AVOID

These foods are the real villains. They can lead to excess weight gain, bloating, cellulite, erratic blood sugar levels and cravings. When you stop eating these foods, for the first few days you may find you experience headaches and cravings, but persevere and you will soon feel more energized, vibrant, healthy, and awake. Your skin will improve, too.

- White bread
- White pasta
- White rice
- Refined cereals
- Sugar
- Cakes
- Pastries
- Croissants
- Cookies
- Chocolate
- Candy
- Ice cream
- Chips
- Artificial flavorings, preservatives, and additives
- Saturated fats—avoid fried or processed foods
- Trans fats—avoid foods labeled hydrogenated fats or oil
- Ready meals
- Tea
- Coffee
- Carbonated drinks
- Fruit concentrate
- Alcohol

DIET MAINTENANCE PLAN

When you have finished the 6 weeks of diet and exercise, you will not only be seeing your results but feeling them too! Don't worry if you still have a little way to go before your stomach is as toned as you would like it to be: you have already done really well in getting this far, and by staying within the Waistline Diet Plan guidelines you will reach your goal. You have put in a lot of effort and commitment so far; keep up the good work with the Diet Maintenance Plan.

A PLAN FOR LIFE

If your weight is now where you want it to be, all you have to do is maintain it. If it's not quite there yet, then simply repeat the Waistline Diet Plan again.

You can use the Waistline Diet Plan as the basis for maintaining your ideal weight rather than losing any more. Start by simply adding in a few extras: for example, increase your portion of porridge for breakfast, introduce lowfat rather than skim milk or have an extra smoothie during the day. You can also substitute in some favorite healthy recipes of your own.

Take care not to overdo the extras, particularly in the early days. You will find that if you re-introduce alcohol, for example, this will quickly increase your calorie intake and you may put on weight.

Maintaining the new you means changes for life. It really won't be as hard as you imagine, so believe in yourself and enjoy the journey.

KEEPING GOING

It can be all too easy to slip back into old habits, so keep reminding yourself that healthy eating is part of your new regime. Fortunately, there are lots of ways of maintaining your new look and healthy lifestyle.

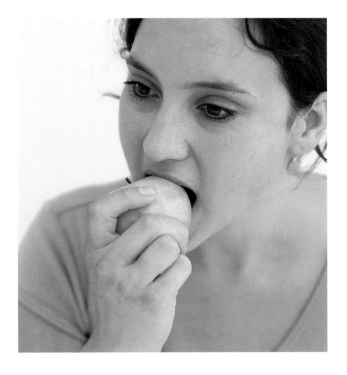

- Keep a food diary and record everything you eat and drink. Don't cheat: the only person who stands to lose is you.
- Eat regular small, healthy meals and snacks every day.
- Eat breakfast, every day: you will be healthier and less likely to consume extra calories during the day.
- Continue to eat a healthy, balanced diet.
- Only eat refined foods occasionally.
- Drink plenty of water daily.
- Prepare your lunch in advance.
- Write a shopping list and stick to it.
- Get outside in the fresh air every day, even if it is just for a short walk.
- Make some time to exercise every day—as little as 10 minutes will still be beneficial.
- Reduce stress levels—the hormone cortisol needs to be kept in check (see page 12).
- Learn to breathe properly: it helps to reduce stress, lowers blood pressure, and encourages weight loss.

Days 1 and 22

BREAKFAST

⅔ cup apple juice

Bowl of porridge
Make with ¾ cup rolled oats and ¾ cup skim or soy milk, using 2 chopped, dried apricots or prunes to sweeten.

OR

⅔ cup pineapple juice

Large bowl of exotic fruit and 1 toasted bagel
Use fresh mango, pineapple, and papaya, with a dash of orange juice and a sprinkling of sunflower seeds. Spread the bagel with 1 tablespoon lowfat cream cheese.

MID-MORNING SNACK

Handful of white grapes or an apple

LUNCH

2 hard-cooked eggs and salad
Season the eggs with paprika and use mixed salad leaves (arugula, baby spinach, radicchio) topped with 6 cherry tomatoes and dressed with 1 teaspoon olive oil mixed with lemon juice.

OR

Vegetable kebabs
Make up 2 skewers per person with seasoned tofu, mushrooms, sweet peppers, zucchini, and onion, with a drizzle of olive oil. Broil for 5–10 minutes.

Strawberries or a pear

MID-AFTERNOON SNACK

2 oatcakes, topped with 1 teaspoon hummus

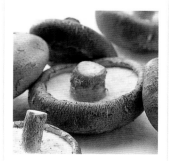

TIP OF THE DAY

From the day you begin the Waistline Diet Plan, keep a diary of how you feel. You may be surprised at how much healthier and more alert you are, and how your tastes for different foods change over the weeks.

DINNER

Seared tuna with lemony salsa
(see recipe)

OR

6–8 vegetarian nuggets per person with Vietnamese salad
Mix a salad of sliced carrots, scallions, and Chinese cabbage, bean sprouts and chopped mint. Toss with a dressing of ½ tablespoon each sunflower oil, rice vinegar, and light soy sauce and ½ teaspoon Thai fish sauce per person.

Berries with yogurt
For each person, spoon 2–3 tablespoons lowfat plain yogurt over a handful of strawberries, blueberries, blackberries, and raspberries.

Seared Tuna with Lemony Salsa

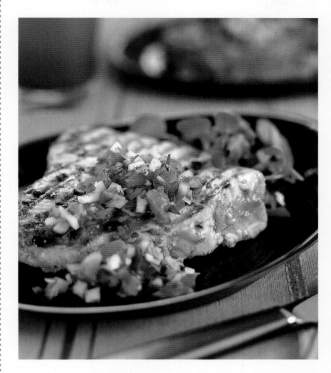

1 Place the tuna steaks on a cutting board and rub half the garlic into one side of the steaks, followed by half the ground fennel seeds and one of the chilies. Turn the steaks over and repeat the process on the other side with the remaining garlic, fennel, and chili.

2 Place the fish in a shallow container and pour over the olive oil and lemon juice. Cover and allow to marinate for 1 hour.

3 Meanwhile, make the salsa. Combine all the ingredients together in a bowl and then put it to one side to let the flavors develop.

4 Preheat a griddle or barbecue grill to very hot and sear the tuna for 1–2 minutes on each side. The tuna should be pink in the middle when it is served. If you prefer it cooked through, cook for an additional 2 minutes on each side.

5 Serve the tuna hot with the salsa, garnished with watercress leaves and the lemon zest. Accompany the tuna with mixed salad leaves (lettuce, chicory, watercress).

Preparation time: 30 minutes, plus marinating
Cooking time: 5 minutes
Serves 4

4 tuna steaks, about 13 oz in total, cut about ¾ in thick
3 garlic cloves, finely chopped
1 teaspoon fennel seeds, finely ground
2 small dried red chilies, crumbled
1 tablespoon olive oil
4 tablespoons lemon juice

Salsa
8 oz beefsteak tomatoes, skinned, seeded, and finely chopped
1 small red onion, finely chopped
1 garlic clove, crushed
½ green chili, seeded, and chopped
2 tablespoons lemon juice
grated zest from 1 unwaxed lemon
¼ cup cilantro leaves, chopped
pinch of superfine sugar

To garnish
handful of watercress leaves
grated zest from 1 unwaxed lemon

NUTRITION

- Carbohydrate 5 g
- Fat 8 g
- Protein 25 g
- Energy 190 kcal (799 kJ)

Days 2 and 23

BREAKFAST

Mango and banana smoothie
Blend the flesh of 1 mango and 1 banana with ⅔ cup skim milk, and add crushed ice.

OR

⅔ cup orange juice

Yogurt with granola
Spoon 2 heaping tablespoons sugar-free granola into ⅔ cup lowfat fruit yogurt.

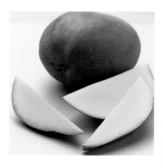

MID-MORNING SNACK

6 dried apricots or 3 fresh dates

LUNCH

Bean curry
Serves 2

Heat 2 teaspoons sunflower oil, add 1 teaspoon cumin seeds and let them pop for a few seconds. Stir in 1 tablespoon tomato paste, 1 teaspoon each ground spices (turmeric, coriander, and cumin) and 2 teaspoons garam masala. Blend over a low heat. Mix in a 13 oz can kidney beans, 2 sliced scallions, and 2 tablespoons chopped cilantro leaves. Season with pepper and serve with brown rice.

OR

Tortillas
Make a salsa by combining 1½ tablespoons ricotta cheese, ½ red onion, 1 tomato, ¼ green chili, and 1 tablespoon cilantro, all finely chopped. Brush 2 flour tortillas with a little olive oil, then cook very briefly on each side on a griddle. Fill each tortilla with the salsa and serve with mixed salad leaves.

MID-AFTERNOON SNACK

2 rice cakes spread thinly with peanut butter

TIP OF THE DAY

Legumes such as kidney beans and split red lentils are high in soluble fiber, which helps to control glucose levels and regulate your appetite. They are also thought to lower blood cholesterol. Another reason to include a daily serving of these foods is that they contain phytoestrogens, which balance falling levels of estrogen—common around the time of the menopause and a major cause of weight gain.

Jamaican Chicken with Sweet Potato Wedges

DINNER

Jamaican chicken with sweet potato wedges
(see recipe)

OR

Red lentil dhal
Serves 4

Soak 1 cup red lentils in warm water. Fry 1 onion, 2 cloves garlic, ½ in fresh ginger root and 2 chilies, all chopped, for 3–5 minutes. Stir in 4 chopped tomatoes and soften. Add ½ teaspoon ground turmeric and 1½ teaspoons garam masala. Cover and simmer for 5 minutes. Add the drained lentils with 2 cups hot water and cook for 15–20 minutes. Add salt, 4 tablespoons lemon juice, and chopped cilantro. Serve with brown rice.

Honeyed figs
Serves 4

Halve 8 fresh figs, drizzle with honey and broil for 2–3 minutes. Garnish with chopped flat-leaf parsley and serve with raspberries and 1 slice of lowfat goat cheese per person.

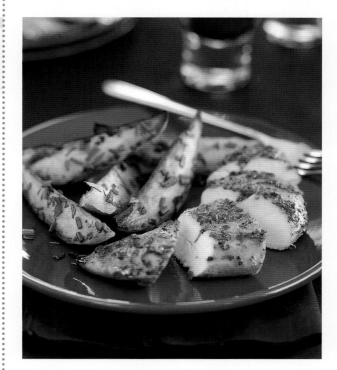

Preparation time:
20 minutes
Cooking time:
35–40 minutes
Serves 4

4 skinless chicken breast fillets, about 1 lb in total

Jerk seasoning
8–10 allspice berries, crushed
2 scallions, green part only, sliced
4 garlic cloves, crushed
(½ in fresh ginger root, peeled and shredded
pinch of grated nutmeg
2 pinches of ground cinnamon
1 teaspoon thyme
1–2 Scotch Bonnet chilies, seeded and finely chopped
2 tablespoons soy sauce
juice of 2 limes

Sweet potato wedges
2 orange-fleshed sweet potatoes, about 1½ lb in total, unpeeled
1 tablespoon olive oil
2 tablespoons chopped parsley
2 tablespoons chopped chives

1 Make the jerk seasoning. Mix the allspice berries with the scallions and pound until well mixed. Add the garlic, ginger, nutmeg, cinnamon, thyme, and chilies. Stir in the soy sauce and lime juice and mix well. If necessary, add a little water to bind.

2 Score the chicken breasts on both sides and rub in the seasoning. Bake the chicken in a preheated oven, 375ºF, for 30–40 minutes until it is crusty on the outside.

3 Meanwhile, put the sweet potatoes in cold water and bring to a boil. Cook the potatoes for 8–10 minutes until parboiled, drain and allow to cool. Remove the skins and cut into wedges.

4 Heat the oil in a nonstick pan and fry the wedges for about 10 minutes until they are browned on both sides. Sprinkle with the parsley and chives and serve with the cooked chicken cut into thick slices and mixed salad leaves (arugula, lettuce, chicory).

NUTRITION

- Carbohydrate 40 g
- Fat 7 g
- Protein 31 g
- Energy 343 kcal (1452 kJ)

Days 3 and 24

BREAKFAST

⅔ cup vegetable juice

Bowl of porridge
Make with ¾ cup rolled oats and ¾ cup skim or soy milk, using 1 grated apple to sweeten.

OR

½ grapefruit

Soft-cooked egg and 1 slice of wholegrain toast spread thinly with olive oil spread

MID-MORNING SNACK

Small handful of nuts and seeds
Choose from almonds, Brazil nuts, hazelnuts, cashew nuts, pumpkin seeds, sunflower seeds, or flax seeds.

LUNCH

Watercress soup
Serves 4

Fry 1 chopped onion until soft, add 2½ cups watercress, 2½ cups vegetable stock, salt and pepper, and 2 tablespoons brown rice. Simmer until the rice is tender, then puree. Stir in 1¼ cups lowfat milk and ⅔ cup lowfat plain yogurt and reheat gently. Serve with 1 slice wholegrain or rye bread.

OR

Omelet and salad
Make with 2 eggs and use mixed salad leaves (arugula, baby spinach, watercress), drizzled with lemon juice and olive oil.

MID-AFTERNOON SNACK

Apple, pear, or nectarine

TIP OF THE DAY

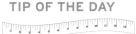

Flax seeds are high in omega-3 oils. They also contain phytoestrogens, which may help combat menopausal hot flashes and offer protection against breast cancer.

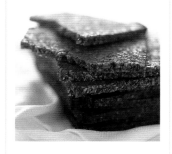

DINNER

Broiled sea bass
(see recipe)

OR

Mushroom stroganoff
Serves 4

Fry 1 sliced onion in 1½ tablespoons olive oil until lightly browned. Add 5 cups sliced mushrooms and 2 finely chopped garlic cloves. Cook for 4 minutes, stir in 2 teaspoons paprika and cook for 1 minute. Add 6 tablespoons vodka. When bubbling, flame with a match and stand well back. Once the flames subside, stir in 1¾ cups vegetable stock, a pinch each ground mace and ground cinnamon, and salt and pepper. Simmer for 4 minutes. Add 2 cups sliced wild mushrooms and cook for 2 minutes. Stir in 2 tablespoons lowfat sour cream.

2 kiwifruit or 3 fresh apricots per person

Broiled Sea Bass

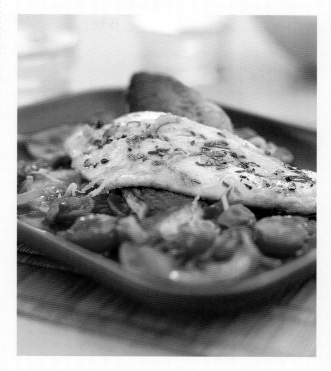

1 Heat the oil in a skillet, add the onion and fry for 5 minutes until softened and lightly browned. Add the tomatoes, saffron (if using), wine, and stock and stir in the lemon zest and a little salt and pepper. Bring to a boil and cook for 2 minutes.

2 Pour the mixture into the base of a foil-lined broiler pan, add the lemon slices and set aside until ready to complete.

3 Arrange the fish fillets, skin side uppermost, on top of the tomatoes. Use a teaspoon to scoop some of the juices over the skin, then sprinkle with salt and pepper and the fennel seeds.

4 Cook under a preheated broiler for 5–6 minutes until the skin is crispy and the fish flakes easily when pressed with a knife. Transfer to serving plates and sprinkle with basil or oregano leaves, if desired. Serve with steamed green vegetables (snow peas, zucchini, broccoli).

Preparation time:
15 minutes
Cooking time: 12–13 minutes
Serves 6

1 tablespoon olive oil
1 onion, finely chopped
10 oz cherry tomatoes, halved
2 large pinches of saffron threads (optional)
⅔ cup dry white wine
½ cup fish stock
grated zest of 1 lemon, the rest halved and thinly sliced
12 small sea bass fillets, about 3–4 oz each, rinsed in cold water
1 teaspoon fennel seeds
salt and pepper
basil or oregano leaves, to garnish (optional)

NUTRITION

- Carbohydrate 4 g
- Fat 7 g
- Protein 39 g
- Energy 252 kcal (1057 kJ)

Days 4 and 25

BREAKFAST	MID-MORNING SNACK	LUNCH	MID-AFTERNOON SNACK
⅔ cup apple juice **Bowl of granola** Make with 1 cup sugar-free granola and ¾ cup skim or soy milk, using 1 sliced banana to sweeten. OR **⅔ cup apple or orange juice** **Exotic fruit salad** Use melon, pineapple, and mango and add 2 tablespoons lowfat plain yogurt.	**Vegetable crudités with hummus** Use a handful of chopped, raw vegetables (carrots, cucumber, sweet peppers, celery, cherry tomatoes) and 2 tablespoons hummus.	**Ricotta, smoked salmon, and artichoke wrap** **(see recipe)** OR **Whole-wheat pita with turkey salad** Fill a pita with tomatoes, lettuce, celery, cucumber, chopped scallions, and a slice of lean turkey breast, plus 1 tablespoon lowfat plain yogurt as dressing. **Pear or apple**	**2 rice cakes spread thinly with tahini or cottage cheese**

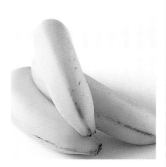

TIP OF THE DAY

Low serotonin levels are linked to depression and weight gain. Turkey, like bananas, is naturally high in serotonin.

DINNER

Peppered steak
Serves 2

Trim the fat from 2 thick-cut porterhouse steaks (1 lb in total) and rub with crushed peppercorns and salt. Mix 1 cup yogurt and 1 crushed garlic clove, add salt and pepper and toss with salad leaves and 1 sliced red onion. Fry the steaks in 1 tablespoon olive oil for 2 minutes. Turn over and cook for 2–5 minutes. Serve with the salad and roasted sweet potatoes.

OR

Sizzling tofu
Serves 2

Marinate 4 oz tofu slices in sesame oil and soy sauce. Dry-fry some sesame seeds, place in a dish and pour the tofu marinade over them. Broil the tofu. Stir-fry ½ in fresh ginger root, 1 garlic clove, 1 shallot, and 8 oz bok choy, all chopped, in 1 tablespoon sunflower oil. Mix in ½ tablespoon each rice vinegar and soy sauce and the sesame seeds. Serve with the tofu.

1 melon slice per person

Ricotta, Smoked Salmon, and Artichoke Wrap

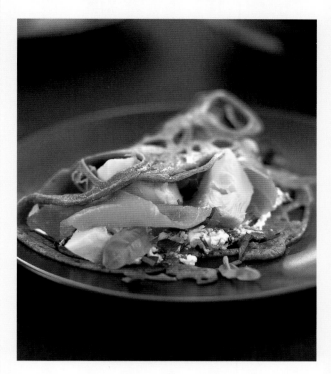

Preparation time:
20 minutes
Cooking time: 15 minutes
Serves 6

Batter
1 cup buckwheat flour
1 egg
1 cup lowfat milk

Filling
½ cup ricotta cheese
3 tablespoons chopped parsley or parsley and basil mixed, plus extra basil leaves to garnish
1 small garlic clove, crushed (optional)
grated zest of ½ lemon and juice of 1 lemon
2 tablespoons sunflower oil
8 oz smoked salmon, sliced
13 oz can artichoke hearts, drained and quartered
salt and pepper

1 Make the batter. Put the flour, egg, a little of the milk and some salt into a bowl and whisk until smooth. Gradually whisk in the remaining milk.

2 Make the filling. Mix the ricotta with the herbs, garlic (if using) and lemon zest and season gently.

3 Heat a little of the oil in a nonstick skillet. When it is hot pour the excess into a small, heatproof bowl. Drizzle in 3 tablespoons of the batter to make lacy crêpes about 18 cm (7 in) in diameter, then cook until the underside is browned. Loosen with a palette knife, turn over and cook the other side in the same way. Lift the crêpe out on to a plate and keep warm. Make 5 more in the same way, adding more oil if needed.

4 Arrange each crêpe on a serving plate, divide the ricotta filling among them and top with strips of smoked salmon and artichoke quarters. Drizzle with lemon juice and sprinkle with pepper. Fold the crêpes over the filling and garnish with some extra chopped herbs.

NUTRITION

- Carbohydrate 19 g
- Fat 10 g
- Protein 19 g
- Energy 229 kcal (958 kJ)

Days 5 and 26

BREAKFAST

Strawberry and raspberry smoothie
Blend together ½ banana, 3 strawberries, 3 raspberries, 1 tablespoon lowfat plain yogurt and ⅔ cup skim or soy milk.

OR

¾ cup apple juice

Soft-cooked egg and 1 slice of wholegrain bread

MID-MORNING SNACK

Handful of white grapes or an apple

LUNCH

Miso broth
Serves 6

Simmer the following for 5 minutes: the white parts of 4 thinly sliced scallions, ¾ in fresh ginger root, finely chopped, 1 sliced red chili, 6 cups fish or vegetable stock, 3 tablespoons chilled miso, 2 tablespoons mirin (Japanese cooking wine), 1 tablespoon soy sauce. Then add the green parts of the scallions, 4 oz bok choy, 2 tablespoons chopped cilantro and 5 oz cooked shrimp. Cook until the bok choy has just wilted.

OR

Small baked potato or sweet potato with ½ cup cottage cheese or tuna.

MID-AFTERNOON SNACK

Oven-baked crunchy chickpeas
Serves 2

Mix together the contents of a 5 oz can chickpeas, drained and rinsed, 1 teaspoon olive oil, and a pinch each of rock salt, ground cumin, chili powder, and ground coriander. Place the mix on a baking sheet and bake in a preheated oven, 400°F, for 10–15 minutes until golden. Allow to cool before serving.

TIP OF THE DAY

Keep your refrigerator stocked up. This will help you to avoid snacking on unhealthy foods.

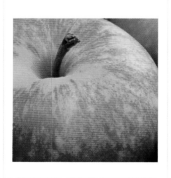

DINNER

Spanish fish stew
(see recipe)

OR

Mediterranean peppers
Serves 4

Put 4 halved bell peppers in an ovenproof dish and fill with 24 halved cherry tomatoes, 2 sliced garlic cloves, 2½ tablespoons capers, and some torn basil leaves. Drizzle with olive oil and season with salt and pepper. Pour some water into the base of the dish, cover with foil, and cook in a preheated oven, 350°F, for 20 minutes. Remove the foil, reduce to 300°F, and bake for 40 minutes. Garnish with more torn basil and serve with salad leaves.

Broiled pineapple and plum sauce
Serves 4

Simmer 14 oz diced plums, 3 star anise, and a pinch each ground chili and cinnamon with 6 tablespoons water until soft. Broil the pineapple slices until lightly browned. Serve with the plum sauce.

Spanish Fish Stew

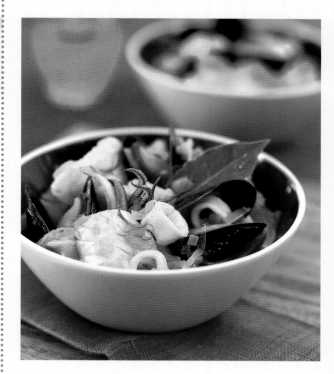

Preparation time:
30 minutes
Cooking time: 24 minutes
Serves 4

1 tablespoon olive oil
1 large onion, finely chopped
2 garlic cloves, finely chopped
½ teaspoon pimentón (smoked paprika)
1 lb tomatoes, skinned and chopped
1 red sweet pepper, cored, seeded and diced
¾ cup fish stock
⅔ cup dry white wine
2 large pinches of saffron threads
4 small bay leaves
1 lb fresh mussels, soaked in cold water
7 oz cleaned calamari, rinsed in cold water
12 oz cod loin, skinned
salt and pepper

1 Heat the oil in a large saucepan, add the onion and fry for 5 minutes until softened and just beginning to brown. Stir in the garlic and pimentón and cook for 1 minute.

2 Mix in the tomatoes, red pepper, fish stock, wine, and saffron. Add the bay leaves, season to taste with salt and pepper and bring to a boil. Cover and simmer gently for 10 minutes. Set aside until needed.

3 Discard any mussels that are open or cracked. Scrub the shells with a nailbrush, remove any barnacles and pull off the hairy tuft-like beard. Return the mussels to a bowl of clean water. Separate the calamari tubes from the tentacles and slice the tubes. Cut the cod into cubes.

4 Reheat the tomato sauce if necessary, add the cod and the calamari slices and cook for 2 minutes. Add the mussels, cover and cook for 4 minutes. Add the calamari tentacles and cook for 2 minutes until cooked through and all the mussels have opened. Gently stir and spoon into bowls to serve.

NUTRITION

- Carbohydrate 11 g
- Fat 5 g
- Protein 32 g
- Energy 240 kcal (1009 kJ)

Days 6 and 27

BREAKFAST

MID-MORNING SNACK

LUNCH

MID-AFTERNOON SNACK

¾ cup pomegranate juice

Fresh fruit compote
Use kiwifruit, pineapple, papaya, and mango.
Top with 2 tablespoons lowfat plain yogurt and a sprinkling of sunflower seeds.

OR

⅔ cup chilled tomato juice

Savory bagel
Spread the bagel with 1 tablespoon lowfat cream cheese and top with 1 oz smoked salmon or wafer-thin honey-roast ham.

Nectarine or peach

Chicken salad Thai style
(see recipe)

OR

Chickpea and olive salad
Serves 4

Stir together the contents of a drained 8 oz can chickpeas, ⅓ cup black olives, ½ chopped red onion, 5 oz chopped tomatoes, and 3 tablespoons chopped flat-leaf parsley. Toss with a mixed dressing of 1 crushed garlic clove, ½ cup lowfat plain yogurt and the juice of ½ lime, seasoned with pepper. Serve on a bed of watercress.

⅔ cup lowfat plain yogurt with 1 teaspoon honey

1 slice of malt loaf

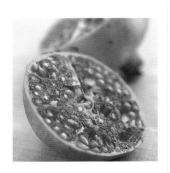

TIP OF THE DAY

Pomegranates are packed with vitamins C and E and folic acid. They contain 3 times the antioxidant levels of tea or red wine. A glass of pomegranate juice per day can help to reduce the risk of cardiovascular disease.

DINNER

Broiled/poached salmon

Serve a 5 oz salmon steak per person with steamed vegetables.

OR

Stir-fried noodles
Serves 4

Cook 8 oz thread egg noodles. Stir-fry 1 onion and ½ in fresh ginger root, both chopped, in 1 tablespoon groundnut oil for 2–3 minutes. Add 7 oz chopped mushrooms and cook for 1–2 minutes. Add 1¼ cups bean sprouts, 2 sliced red sweet peppers, 1 tablespoon plum sauce, 2 tablespoons soy sauce, and 6 sliced scallions, and cook for a few minutes. Mix in the noodles.

Baked bananas

Slice 1 banana per person lengthwise and wrap in foil with 1 tablespoon water, ½ tablespoon honey, ½ teaspoon lemon juice, 1½ tablespoons raisins, and a pinch of cinnamon. Bake in a preheated oven, 400°F, for 10 minutes.

Chicken Salad Thai Style

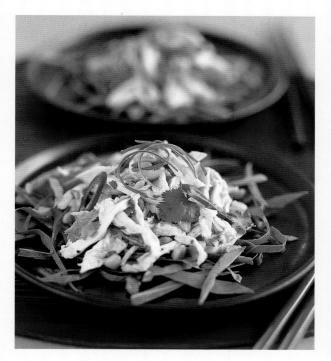

Preparation time:
10 minutes
Cooking time:
15–20 minutes
Serves 4

5 oz cooked chicken breast, shredded
3 tablespoons cilantro leaves
5 oz bok choy, shredded

Dressing
1 tablespoon groundnut oil
1 tablespoon Thai fish sauce
juice of 1 lime
juice of 1 small orange
1 garlic clove, crushed
3 tablespoons roughly chopped basil leaves
pepper

To garnish
2 scallions, green stems only, shredded lengthwise
1 plump red chili, seeded and sliced diagonally

1 Make the dressing by shaking all the ingredients together in a screw-top jar.

2 Mix the chicken with the cilantro leaves and then stir in the dressing.

3 Line a serving dish with the bok choy, spoon the dressed chicken on top and serve chilled, garnished with scallion shreds and red chili slices.

NUTRITION

- Carbohydrate 4 g
- Fat 7 g
- Protein 16 g
- Energy 144 kcal (604 kJ)

Days 7 and 28

BREAKFAST

Carrot and apple juice
Juice together 3 carrots, 2 apples, and 2 sticks of celery.

Bowl of granola
Make with 1 cup sugar-free granola and ¾ cup skim or soy milk or 3 tablespoons lowfat plain yogurt, using 1 grated apple to sweeten.

OR

⅔ cup apple juice

2 scrambled eggs and 1 slice of wholegrain toast

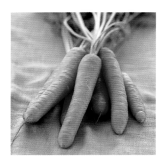

MID-MORNING SNACK

6 dried apricots or 6 Brazil nuts

LUNCH

Bulgar wheat salad
Serves 2

Soak 1 cup bulgar wheat for 30 minutes, then drain and squeeze dry. Add 4 sliced plums, 1 crushed garlic clove, 1 finely chopped red onion, a handful each chopped parsley and mint, 2 tablespoons olive oil, and 4 tablespoons lemon juice. Add salt and pepper, and refrigerate for at least 30 minutes. Serve with 4 tablespoons lowfat yogurt, mixed with 1 crushed garlic clove, ½ teaspoon each cayenne pepper and tomato paste and some finely chopped chives.

OR

Whole-wheat tuna pita
Fill a pita with the drained contents of a 6½ oz can tuna, mixed salad leaves (radicchio, chicory, arugula) and some chopped cherry tomatoes, red onion, and parsley or cilantro. Add a squeeze of lemon juice, 1 tablespoon lowfat plain yogurt, and some chopped mint.

MID-AFTERNOON SNACK

2 pieces of fruit
Choose from apple, nectarine, satsuma, pear, or a small handful of grapes.

TIP OF THE DAY

If you are eating out in a restaurant, go for the healthy option. Ask for the sauce to be served on the side and for there to be no dressing on salad and vegetables.

DINNER

Herby lamb
(see recipe)

OR

Lentil pilaf
Serves 4

Sauté 1 chopped garlic clove and 1 chopped bunch scallions in 1 tablespoon olive oil until soft. Add $\frac{1}{2}$ cup lentils, $\frac{1}{4}$ cup each brown rice and wild rice, and $2\frac{1}{2}$ cups vegetable stock. Bring to a boil, then turn down the heat and simmer until nearly all the stock has gone. Add 1 tablespoon each chopped almonds and chopped thyme. Serve with mixed green leaves (baby spinach, watercress, radicchio).

**1 sliced papaya
per person**

Herby Lamb

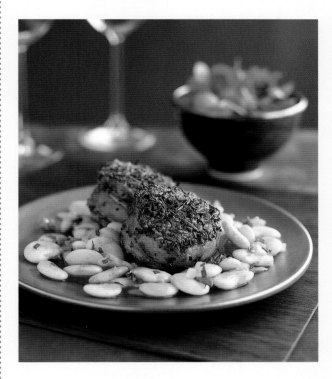

1 Mix together all the chopped herbs in a bowl. Spread mustard on both sides of each noisette and dip the meat into the herb mixture. Press the herbs firmly to the mustard. Chill the lamb in the refrigerator until you are ready to cook.

2 Make the tangy lima beans. Heat the oil in a skillet and fry the onion until it has softened. Add the remainder of the ingredients to the skillet and cook gently for 5 minutes.

3 Preheat the broiler to hot and cook the lamb noisettes for about 4 minutes each side. The lamb should be cooked but still retain a slight pink color.

4 Serve the lamb immediately, surrounded by the tangy lima beans. Accompany with steamed green vegetables (zucchini, broccoli, cabbage, cauliflower).

Preparation time:
10 minutes
Cooking time:
15–20 minutes
Serves 4

**2 tablespoons finely
    chopped mint**
**1 tablespoon finely chopped
    thyme**
**1 tablespoon finely chopped
    oregano**
**$\frac{1}{2}$ tablespoon finely chopped
    rosemary**
**4 teaspoons wholegrain
    mustard**
**4 lamb noisettes, about
    4 oz each**

Tangy lima beans
2 teaspoons sunflower oil
1 medium onion, chopped
**$1\frac{1}{2}$ cups cooked lima beans
    or drained canned beans**
1 tablespoon tomato paste
**3 tablespoons pineapple
    juice**
2 tablespoons lemon juice
**a few drops of Tabasco
    sauce**
pepper

NUTRITION

- Carbohydrate 14 g
- Fat 14 g
- Protein 32 g
- Energy 305 kcal (1280 kJ)

Days 8 and 29

BREAKFAST	MID-MORNING SNACK	LUNCH	MID-AFTERNOON SNACK
⅔ cup orange juice	**Small handful of toasted nuts**	**Whole-wheat pita filled with 4 oz smoked trout and some watercress**	**2 oatcakes topped with 2 tablespoons lowfat cottage cheese**
Large fresh fruit salad Use apple, pear, grapes, and kiwifruit. Top with 2 tablespoons lowfat plain yogurt and a sprinkling of sunflower and flax seeds.	Broil almonds, cashew nuts, or walnuts, or a mixture of these, for 5–7 minutes.	OR	
OR		**Vietnamese vegetable spring rolls** (see recipe)	
⅔ cup apple juice		**⅔ cup lowfat fruit yogurt per person**	
Bowl of wholegrain cereal Make with 2 cups wholegrain cereal and ⅔ cup skim or soy milk.			

TIP OF THE DAY

Nuts are high in essential omega-3 and omega-6 oils. Full of vitamins and minerals, they help you to burn fat by speeding up your metabolism. The secret is not to eat too many of them!

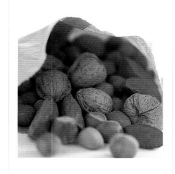

DINNER

Broiled halibut
Serves 4

Brush 4 halibut steaks
(1¼ lb total) with olive oil,
season with salt and pepper,
and broil until cooked.
Stir-fry 1 teaspoon crushed
fresh ginger root and
¼ teaspoon fennel seeds
in 2 tablespoons olive oil
for a few seconds. Add
1 lb broccoli florets, 3
tablespoons soy sauce, and
pepper, and stir-fry until just
cooked. Serve with the fish.

OR

Fruity couscous
Serves 4

Swell 1 cup couscous in hot
vegetable stock. Add
1 stir-fried chopped red
onion and red sweet pepper,
¼ cup each chopped
parsley, basil, and mint, the
juice and zest of 1 lime, a
pinch of ground cinnamon,
⅓ cup chopped dried
apricots, and ¼ cup toasted
slivered almonds. Serve
with mixed salad leaves.

**6 stewed prunes or
2 plums per person**

Vietnamese vegetable spring rolls

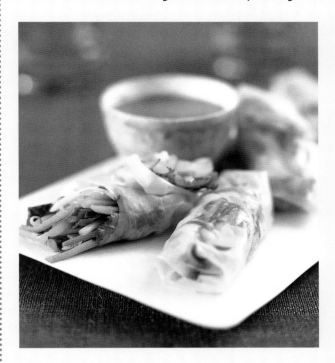

**Preparation time:
30 minutes
Cooking time: 5 minutes
Serves 4**

**7 oz bok choy
2 tablespoons sunflower oil
4 oz sweet potato, cut into
   matchstick strips
4 oz carrot, cut into
   matchstick strips
½ bunch of scallions, cut
   into matchstick strips
½ cup bean sprouts, rinsed
   and drained
2 garlic cloves, finely
   chopped
¾ in piece of fresh ginger
   root, peeled and finely
   chopped
8 rice pancakes
bunch of cilantro**

Sauce
**4 ripe red plums, about
   8 oz in total
2 tablespoons water
1 tablespoon soy sauce
made-up wasabi (Japanese
   horseradish sauce),
   to taste
1 tablespoon superfine sugar**

1 Cut the leaves from the bok choy and slice the stems into
thin matchstick strips. Heat 1 tablespoon of the oil in a wok
or large skillet, add the sweet potato and carrot and stir-fry
for 2 minutes. Add the scallions and bok choy stems and
cook for 1 minute. Mix in the bean sprouts, garlic, and
ginger and cook for 1 minute. Transfer to a bowl.

2 Heat the remaining oil in the pan, add the bok choy
leaves and cook for 2–3 minutes until just wilted.

3 Dip a rice pancake into a bowl of hot water and leave for
20–30 seconds until softened. Lift out and place on a dish
towel. Top with a bok choy leaf, one-eighth of the vegetable
mixture, and 2 stems of cilantro. Fold in the pancake edges
and roll up tightly, repeating to make 8 pancakes in all.
Cover with plastic wrap and set aside. Serve within 1 hour.

4 Meanwhile, make the sauce. Pit and chop the plums.
Place in a small saucepan with the water, cover and cook
for 5 minutes until softened. Puree the plums with the soy
sauce, then mix in the wasabi and sugar to taste.

5 Garnish the pancakes with the remaining sprigs of
cilantro and serve with small bowls of the sauce.

NUTRITION

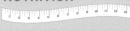

- Carbohydrate 27 g
- Fat 6 g
- Protein 4 g
- Energy 176 kcal (734 kJ)

Days 9 and 30

BREAKFAST

Strawberry and banana smoothie
Blend together 1 banana, 6 strawberries, and ¾ cup chilled skim milk.

OR

⅔ cup orange juice

Bowl of porridge
Make with ¾ cup rolled oats and ¾ cup skim or soy milk, adding 6 chopped strawberries to sweeten.

MID-MORNING SNACK

Vegetable crudités with hummus
Use a handful of chopped, raw vegetables (carrots, cucumber, sweet peppers, celery, cherry tomatoes) and 2 tablespoons hummus.

LUNCH

Avocado salad and 1 slice of rye bread spread thinly with tahini
Slice ½ avocado onto a bed of mixed salad (watercress, baby spinach, radicchio, celery, cherry tomatoes, cucumber).

OR

Filled sandwich of wholegrain bread with olive oil spread
Fill with broiled chicken, mixed salad leaves (baby spinach, lamb's lettuce, radicchio) and some sliced tomato.

Apple or pear

MID-AFTERNOON SNACK

2 rice cakes spread with 2 tablespoons lowfat cream cheese

TIP OF THE DAY

Avocados are a good source of monosaturated fat. This sort of fat is known to maintain levels of good HDL cholesterol, which is associated with a lower risk of cardiovascular disease.

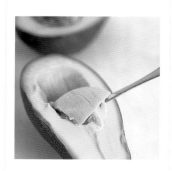

DINNER

Roast pepper and walnut pappardelle
(see recipe)

⅔ cup lowfat fruit yogurt per person

OR

Broiled chicken
Serve a broiled 5 oz chicken breast per person with 4 oz baked sweet potato and a tomato and red onion salad.

Strawberry whip
Blend together 1 banana, 5 strawberries, and 1 tablespoon lowfat plain yogurt per person. Sprinkle with sunflower seeds.

Roast Pepper and Walnut Pappardelle

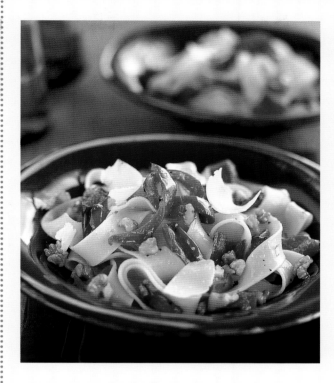

Preparation time:
10–15 minutes
Cooking time: 35 minutes
Serves 4

2 teaspoons olive oil
4 red bell peppers, cored, seeded and sliced
3–4 large garlic cloves, thinly sliced
½ cup chopped walnuts
10 oz fresh egg pappardelle
1 oz Parmesan cheese shavings
salt and pepper

1 Use ½ teaspoon of the olive oil to brush over the peppers. Put the peppers on a baking sheet and roast them in a preheated oven, 450°F, for 20–25 minutes until they are soft and just beginning to blacken.

2 Reserve 4 slices of pepper to use as a garnish and cut the remaining slices into large dice.

3 Heat the remaining olive oil in a large skillet over a medium-low heat, add the sliced garlic but do not let it brown. Add the diced red pepper and stir in the walnuts. Keep warm.

4 Bring a large saucepan of lightly salted water to a boil. Add the pasta, return to a boil and cook for 3–4 minutes or until the pasta is *al dente*. Drain and transfer to a large, warm serving bowl.

5 Toss the pasta well with the garlic, pepper, and walnut mixture. Sprinkle over the Parmesan shavings and garnish with the reserved pepper slices.

NUTRITION

- Carbohydrate 63 g
- Fat 16 g
- Protein 15 g
- Energy 435 kcal (1833 kJ)

Days 10 and 31

BREAKFAST

²⁄₃ cup apple juice

2 large broiled tomatoes on 1 slice of wholegrain toast

OR

²⁄₃ cup pineapple juice

Bagel spread with 1½ tablespoons lowfat cream cheese, with 1 slice lean ham and 1 tomato.

MID-MORNING SNACK

2 pieces of fruit
Choose from apple, pear, orange, peach, or nectarine.

LUNCH

Chicken and bean salad
Serves 2

Mix together 1 tablespoon lemon juice, 1 teaspoon olive oil, and a pinch each of paprika and pepper to make the dressing. Mix together the salad ingredients: 2 oz cooked, sliced chicken breast, ¼ cup cooked kidney beans, ⅓ cup cooked chickpeas; 1 oz each finely sliced, cooked leeks, sliced red sweet pepper, sliced mushrooms. Pour over the dressing and mix well. Serve on a bed of mixed salad leaves (baby spinach, arugula, lettuce).

OR

Tofu and bean salad
Make as above, substituting the chicken with broiled tofu.

MID-AFTERNOON SNACK

Small handful of pumpkin and sunflower seeds

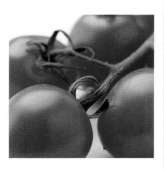

TIP OF THE DAY

Tomatoes are a rich source of vitamins A and C. They also contain lycopene, an antioxidant that has been linked to a reduced risk of breast, pancreatic, and ovarian cancers.

DINNER

Griddled artichokes and fennel
(see recipe)

Serve with a 5 oz pan-fried salmon fillet or tuna steak and ¼ cup brown rice per person.

OR

Serve the artichokes with 4 oz baked tofu and ¼ cup brown rice per person.

Baked pear with almond crumble
Serves 4

Mix ¾ cup whole-wheat flour, ½ cup ground almonds and ⅓ cup brown sugar. Blend in 5 tablespoons butter until the mixture resembles fine bread crumbs. Arrange 4 pears, unpeeled, cored and sliced lengthwise, in 4 tall ovenproof ramekins and drizzle with the juice of 1 lime. Cover with the crumble and sprinkle over 2 tablespoons slivered almonds. Bake in a preheated oven, 425°F, for 20 minutes. Serve warm, topped with lowfat sour cream, if desired.

Griddled Artichokes and Fennel

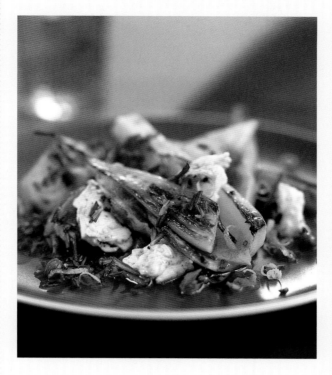

**Preparation time:
15 minutes
Cooking time: 7–8 minutes
Serves 6**

**3 tablespoons olive oil
3 teaspoons finely chopped
 rosemary leaves
7 oz fennel heads, stems
 separated and any large
 pieces halved
13 oz can artichoke hearts,
 drained and halved
4 oz feta cheese, drained
 and crumbled
sprigs of rosemary, to
 garnish**

Dressing
**grated zest and juice of
 1 lemon
2 teaspoons capers, drained
4 teaspoons balsamic
 vinegar
salt and pepper**

1 Put the oil, chopped rosemary, and a little salt and pepper in a plastic bag. Add the fennel and artichoke hearts and shake gently in the bag.

2 Heat a ridged skillet, add the dressed vegetables and cook for 3–4 minutes until the undersides are browned. Turn them over and cook for 2 minutes. Crumble the cheese over the top and place the pan under a preheated broiler for 2 more minutes until the cheese is hot but not melted.

3 Meanwhile, mix the dressing ingredients together with any remaining oil in the plastic bag.

4 Spoon the vegetables onto serving plates and drizzle the dressing over the top. Garnish with extra rosemary leaves torn from the stems.

NUTRITION

- Carbohydrate 3 g
- Fat 9 g
- Protein 5 g
- Energy 109 kcal (454 kJ)

Days 11 and 32

BREAKFAST

⅔ cup orange juice

Bowl of wholegrain cereal
Make with 2 cups wholegrain cereal and ⅓ cup skim or soy milk, adding 3 chopped dried apricots or prunes to sweeten.

OR

⅔ cup apple juice

2 soft-cooked eggs and 1 slice of wholegrain bread spread thinly with olive oil spread

MID-MORNING SNACK

2 rice cakes spread thinly with lowfat cream cheese

LUNCH

Vegetable omelette
Make with 2 eggs and add chopped red sweet pepper, scallion, and zucchini.

OR

Mixed rice and vegetables
Mix ⅓ cup cooked brown and wild rice with 4 oz chopped broiled chicken and some chopped red sweet pepper, scallion, and corn. Mix the juice of ½ lemon, 1 teaspoon olive oil, and black pepper, and pour over the rice.

MID-AFTERNOON SNACK

Fruit smoothie
Blend together 1 kiwifruit, 1 sliced banana, 2 chopped dried apricots, 1 teaspoon honey and 1 cup skim or soy milk, then add 2 tablespoons lowfat plain yogurt.

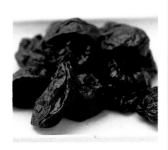

TIP OF THE DAY

Keep a bowl of cherry tomatoes, sliced sweet peppers, and celery, carrot, and cucumber sticks in the fridge, ready for those times when you feel the need to snack.

DINNER

Flaming chicken
Serves 4

Fry 4 chicken breasts, about 5 oz each, and 8 oz halved shallots in 1 tablespoon olive oil until the chicken is browned underneath. Turn it over and add 1 chopped garlic clove, 1 diced apple, and 1 cup sliced mushrooms. Fry until cooked. Spoon 4 tablespoons Calvados over the chicken and flame with a match. Once the flames subside, add 1 cup stock, 1 teaspoon mustard, and thyme. Season and cook for 5 minutes. Serve with steamed vegetables.

OR

Vegetable noodles
Serves 4

Stir-fry 2 chopped sweet peppers, 8 oz each snow peas, sliced mushrooms, and zucchini, and 5 oz baby corn in 2 tablespoons each soy sauce and olive oil for 5 minutes. Add 1¼ lb buckwheat noodles and fry until cooked.

Oriental melon
(see recipe)

Oriental Melon

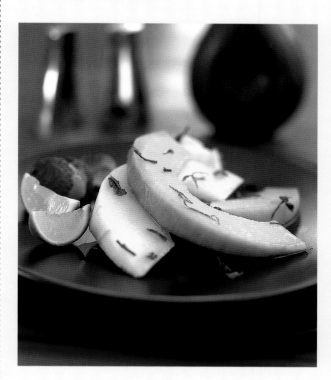

Preparation time:
15 minutes, plus chiling
Cooking time: none
Serves 6

2 orange-flavored green
  teabags
1¼ cups boiling water
1 orange-fleshed cantaloupe
  melon, such as charentais
½ green-fleshed melon, such
  as galia or ogen
½ honeydew melon
2 tablespoons light cane
  sugar
grated zest and juice of
  1 lime

To decorate
lime wedges
6 fresh lychees

1 Put the teabags into a jug and pour the boiling water over them. Allow to infuse for 2 minutes (no longer or it will taste bitter). Lift out the bags, draining them well. Break open one of the bags, remove a few tea leaves and add them to the tea infusion. Allow to cool.

2 Halve the whole melon and scoop out the seeds. Remove the seeds from the other melons. Cut away the skin with a small knife and cut the orange- and green-fleshed melons into long, thin slices. Dice the honeydew melon. Put all the prepared melon into a large, shallow dish.

3 Sprinkle the sugar and lime zest and juice over the melon and pour over the tea. Cover with plastic wrap and chill for 1 hour, or overnight if preferred.

4 Arrange the long melon slices in fan shapes on individual serving plates. Spoon the diced melon to the side of the melon fans and serve each one with lime wedges and a partially peeled lychee.

NUTRITION

- Carbohydrate 20 g
- Fat 0 g
- Protein 2 g
- Energy 83 kcal (353 kJ)

Days 12 and 33

BREAKFAST	MID-MORNING SNACK	LUNCH	MID-AFTERNOON SNACK

¾ cup pineapple juice

2 scrambled eggs and 1 slice of whole-wheat toast spread thinly with olive oil spread

OR

¾ cup pomegranate juice

Bowl of granola
Make with 1 cup sugar-free granola and ⅓ cup skim or soy milk.

Pear and a small handful of pumpkin seeds

Tuna or feta salad
Make with 3 oz fresh or 2½ oz canned tuna or 2 oz feta cheese and mixed salad leaves (baby spinach, watercress, lettuce), bean sprouts, 5 cherry tomatoes, and fresh cilantro and basil leaves. Dress with a little olive oil and cider vinegar

3 oatcakes

OR

Wholegrain turkey sandwich
Spread 2 slices wholegrain bread with 1 teaspoon low-calorie mayonnaise and fill with 5 oz lean turkey breast, lettuce, and sliced tomato.

Pieces of fruit
Choose from 2 kiwifruit, 2 plums, or a pear.

Plum and a small handful of almonds

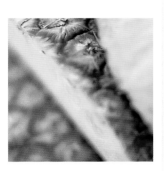

DINNER

Scallops in pancetta with lemon lentils
(see recipe)

OR

Tempeh with lemon lentils
(see recipe)

Substitute the scallops and pancetta with tempeh for a vegetarian option.

⅔ cup lowfat fruit yogurt per person

TIP OF THE DAY

Bromelain enzymes are found in pineapple. They have a powerful anti-inflammatory effect and also improve digestion.

Scallops in Pancetta with Lemon Lentils

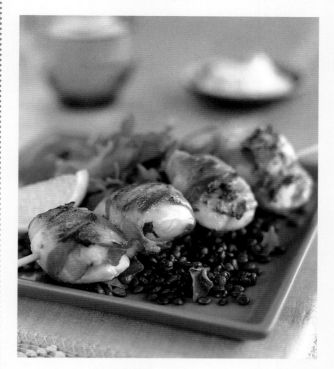

Preparation time:
15 minutes
Cooking time: 45 minutes
Serves 4

16 scallops, about 13 oz in total, roe removed
2 tablespoons chopped oregano leaves
7 oz pancetta, cut into 16 thin slices

Lemon lentils
1 teaspoon olive oil
1 onion, chopped
6 cloves
1 cup Puy lentils, washed
1¾ cups vegetable stock
1¾ cups hot water
4–6 tablespoons lemon juice
pepper

To garnish
mixed salad leaves
1 lemon, cut into 4 wedges
⅔ cup lowfat plain yogurt sprinkled with lemon zest
handful of oregano leaves

1 Prepare the lemon lentils by heating the olive oil in a saucepan over medium to low heat. Add the onion and cook for about 5 minutes, stirring occasionally, until it begins to brown. Add the whole cloves and lentils and cook for 5 minutes.

2 Pour in the vegetable stock and the measurement water and bring to a boil. Simmer gently, uncovered, for 30 minutes until the lentils are tender.

3 Meanwhile, sprinkle the scallops with the chopped oregano and wrap each in a slice of pancetta. Thread 4 scallop parcels onto a skewer. Repeat with the rest of the scallops. Broil the scallops on a barbecue or under a preheated hot broiler for 2–3 minutes each side until they are golden brown.

4 Remove and discard the cloves from the lentils and stir in the lemon juice and pepper. Serve the scallops and lentils garnished with mixed salad leaves, a lemon wedge, and yogurt, and sprinkled with oregano leaves.

NUTRITION

- Carbohydrate 36 g
- Fat 16 g
- Protein 47 g
- Energy 467 kcal (1967 kJ)

Days 13 and 34

BREAKFAST

⅔ cup tomato juice

Bowl of porridge
Make with ¾ cup rolled oats and ¾ cup skim or soy milk, using 1 grated apple to sweeten.

OR

⅔ cup orange juice

Crunchy yogurt
Mix 1 tablespoon each toasted jumbo oats and mixed berries (strawberries, blueberries, blackberries, raspberries) into ⅔ cup lowfat plain yogurt and sprinkle 2 tablespoons mixed seeds (pumpkin, sunflower, sesame) on top.

MID-MORNING SNACK

2 oatcakes spread thinly with peanut butter

LUNCH

Savory bagel
Spread a bagel with 1½ tablespoons lowfat cream cheese and top with 1 oz smoked salmon.

OR

Whole-wheat pita with cottage cheese
Fill a pita with ½ cup cottage cheese, sliced cucumber, and chopped chives.

Orange or mango

MID-AFTERNOON SNACK

Small handful of toasted nuts
Broil almonds, cashew nuts, or walnuts, or a mixture of these, for 5–7 minutes.

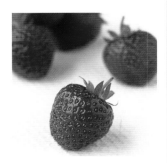

TIP OF THE DAY

Make time to eat! You may have had a long day or need to rush off somewhere, but sitting down and really enjoying your food is important for both your digestive system and your health.

DINNER

Marinated shrimp with zucchini
(see recipe)

OR

Quinoa and rice fluff
Serves 4

Fry 1 chopped onion in 1 tablespoon olive oil until soft, then add ¾ cup each quinoa and brown rice and 2½ cups vegetable stock, cover and simmer until the stock has been absorbed and the rice is soft. Add salt and pepper, juice of 1 lemon, and 1 tablespoon chopped cilantro.

Fresh pineapple
Allow 1 large slice (about 5 oz) per person.

Marinated Shrimp with Zucchini

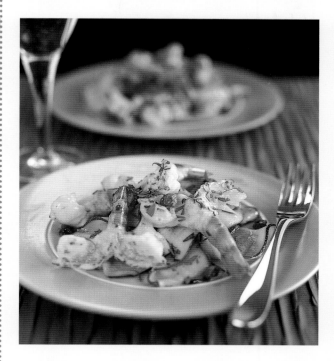

1 Mix together all the marinade ingredients, lightly crushing the capers against the side of the bowl.

2 Spoon two-thirds of the marinade mixture on top of the zucchini ribbons in a large bowl. Marinate for 3–4 hours.

3 Prepare the shrimp. Hold the tail underside up and cut each shrimp in half lengthwise. Pull out any black intestinal thread, rinse, pat dry on paper towels and put in a shallow dish. Alternatively, buy ready-prepared shrimp. Pour the remaining marinade over the shrimp and marinate for 3–4 hours.

4 Place the zucchini in a large pan with their marinade and simmer over a medium-low heat for 3–5 minutes.

5 Broil the shrimp for 3–4 minutes until pink and sizzling, basting with the marinade. Do not overcook them.

6 To serve, pile the zucchini in the center of a warmed dish, top with the shrimp and garnish with chopped parsley. Accompany with ⅓ cup cooked brown rice and steamed broccoli with 1 teaspoon toasted sesame seeds.

Preparation time:
30 minutes, plus marinating
Cooking time: 5 minutes
Serves 4

1 lb zucchini, topped and tailed and sliced into fine ribbons with a vegetable peeler
28 large raw shrimp, peeled but with tails still intact, heads removed
handful of chopped flat-leaf parsley, to garnish

Marinade
large pinch of saffron threads
8 tablespoons lemon juice
6 garlic cloves, roughly chopped
2 tablespoons rice wine vinegar
4 tablespoons olive oil
2 tablespoons drained capers

NUTRITION

- Carbohydrate 6 g
- Fat 12 g
- Protein 12 g
- Energy 175 kcal/728 kJ

Days 14 and 35

BREAKFAST

²⁄₃ cup pomegranate juice

2 large broiled tomatoes on 1 slice of wholegrain toast

OR

²⁄₃ cup orange juice

Savory omelet
Make with 2 eggs and chopped red sweet pepper and mushrooms.

MID-MORNING SNACK

Pear

LUNCH

6 pieces of vegetarian sushi

Exotic fruit salad
Use chopped kiwifruit, pineapple, mango, passion fruit, and papaya. Keep the remainder for your mid-afternoon snack.

OR

Vegetable and bean soup
Serves 6

Gently fry 2 onions, 1 celery stalk, 1 garlic clove and 1 lb 2 oz mixed vegetables (carrots, green beans, broccoli), all chopped, with ½ teaspoon coriander seeds for about 5 minutes. Add 1 chopped sweet potato (about 7 oz), cover the pan and fry gently for 3–4 minutes, until soft. Add 4 cups vegetable stock, 2⅓ cups flageolet beans, and 2 tablespoons chopped fresh herbs. Bring to a boil, then simmer for 10–15 minutes. The soup can be pureed before serving. Serve with a whole-wheat roll, if required.

Pear, peach, or nectarine

MID-AFTERNOON SNACK

Any fruit left over from your lunchtime fruit salad

OR

2 oatcakes and fruit
Choose from mango or peach, or 6 dried apricots or dates.

TIP OF THE DAY

Eggs are more effective for building muscle than any other protein—and more muscle means less body fat.

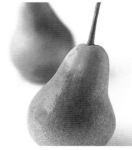

DINNER

Baked salmon fillet

Sprinkle a 5 oz salmon fillet per person with lemon juice and pepper. Wrap in foil and bake in a preheated oven, 400°F, for 12–15 minutes. Serve with sweet potato wedges, broccoli, and carrots.

OR

Pasta with broccoli, olives, and mozzarella
Serves 4

Cook 1 lb broccoli florets until just tender and drain. Fry 1 chopped onion and 1 crushed garlic clove until soft. Add a 13 oz can chopped tomatoes, 1 tablespoon tomato paste, ⅔ cup pitted black olives, the cooked broccoli, and 2 tablespoons thyme. Cook for 3 minutes and season with salt and pepper. Cook 12 oz whole-wheat pasta, toss in the sauce and add 4 oz lowfat buffalo mozzarella, torn into pieces. Serve with a fresh tomato and basil salad.

Baked peaches
(see recipe)

Baked Peaches

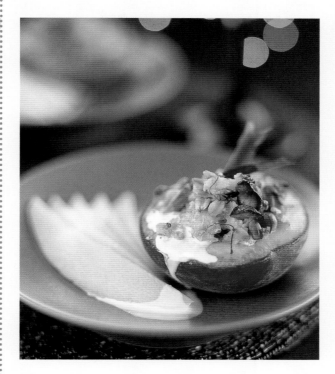

Preparation time: 15 minutes
Cooking time: 15 minutes
Serves 4

2 large, slightly under-ripe peaches, halved and pitted
a few saffron threads
a few drops almond extract
¾ cup crunchy oat cereal
2 tablespoons orange juice
2 in cinnamon stick, broken into 8 pieces

To serve
½ slightly under-ripe mango, thinly sliced
1 teaspoon grated dark chocolate (optional)

1 Scoop some of the flesh out of the peach halves and chop finely. Put the halved peaches, skin side down, in a lightly oiled baking dish.

2 Mix together the chopped peach flesh, saffron, almond extract, oat cereal, and orange juice. Spoon the mixture carefully into the peach halves.

3 Push the cinnamon stick pieces into the peach halves. Bake the peaches uncovered in a preheated oven, 350°F, for 15 minutes.

4 Arrange one peach half on each dessert plate. Serve with mango slices and a sprinkling of grated dark chocolate (if using).

NUTRITION

- Carbohydrate 16 g
- Fat 6 g
- Protein 3 g
- Energy 130 kcal (547 kJ)

Days 15 and 36

BREAKFAST

Fruit smoothie
Blend together ¼ cup lowfat plain yogurt and ½ cup each strawberries, blueberries, and raspberries. Add a few pumpkin seeds and crushed ice if desired.

OR

⅔ cup apple juice

Bowl of granola
Make with 1 cup sugar-free granola and ¾ cup skim or soy milk, using 1 sliced banana to sweeten.

MID-MORNING SNACK

Small handful of grapes or 2 rice cakes lightly spread with goat cheese and 2 cherry tomatoes

LUNCH

Cauliflower cheese soup
Serves 4

Fry 1 finely chopped onion in 1½ tablespoons olive oil until soft. Add 1½ lb cauliflower florets, cover and cook for 5–10 minutes. Stir in 2½ cups vegetable stock and simmer until the cauliflower is tender. Lightly toast some pumpkin seeds. Puree the soup, add ⅓ cup grated strong cheddar cheese and salt and pepper. Reheat until the cheese melts. Garnish with a swirl of yogurt and the toasted pumpkin seeds. Serve with 1 slice of wholegrain or rye bread.

OR

Chicken and rice salad
Mix 4 tablespoons cooked brown rice with a large handful of chopped raw vegetables (cucumber, celery, red sweet pepper, tomatoes, scallions) and 4 oz chopped broiled chicken. Squeeze over 1 teaspoon lemon juice and drizzle with 1 teaspoon olive oil.

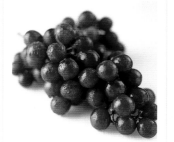

MID-AFTERNOON SNACK

Vegetable crudités with guacamole
Make the guacamole by mashing a ripe avocado into the juice of 1 lime and 1 tablespoon soy sauce. For the crudités, use a handful of chopped, raw vegetables (carrots, cucumber, sweet peppers, celery, cherry tomatoes).

TIP OF THE DAY

Focus on how you want to look and keep that picture in your mind— this is what you are working towards.

DINNER

Bean and lamb roast
(see recipe)

OR

Shrimp stir-fry
Serves 2

Stir-fry 1 garlic clove and a 1 in piece fresh ginger root, both finely chopped, with 4 chopped scallions and ½ teaspoon chili powder for 2 minutes. Add 4 oz snow peas and sliced mushrooms and ½ sliced red sweet pepper, and stir-fry for 4 minutes. Add 1½ cups shredded Chinese cabbage, 1 cup bean sprouts, 7 oz cooked jumbo shrimp, and 1 tablespoon light soy sauce, and heat gently.

Strawberries and yogurt
For each person, spoon 2 tablespoons lowfat plain yogurt over a handful of strawberries, then sprinkle with some toasted sesame and sunflower seeds.

Bean and Lamb Roast

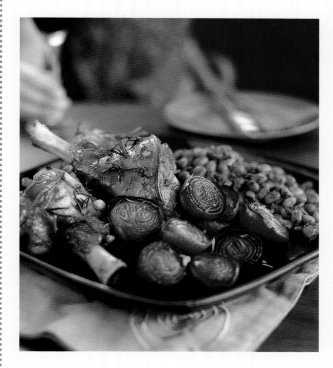

Preparation time:
10 minutes, plus marinating
Cooking time: 2–2½ hours
Serves 4

4 lamb shanks, about
 2½ lb in total, fat removed
4–5 rosemary sprigs
2 garlic cloves, thinly sliced
4 small red onions, halved
3 tablespoons balsamic
 vinegar

Marinade
small bunch of thyme, leaves
 removed from stalks
3 whole cardamom pods
1 bay leaf
pinch of saffron threads
4 tablespoons lemon juice
salt and pepper

Spiced beans
2 teaspoons canola oil
½ teaspoon black mustard
 seeds
½ teaspoon onion seeds
1 tablespoon tomato paste
pinch of ground turmeric
¼–½ teaspoon chili powder
2 x 10 oz cans pinto beans,
 drained
2 tablespoons chopped
 cilantro leaves, plus extra
 to garnish

1 Place the shanks in a roasting pan, make slits in each shank and push in sprigs of rosemary and slices of garlic.

2 Mix the marinade ingredients together. Coat the lamb shanks, cover with foil, and refrigerate for at least 1 hour.

3 Cook the lamb in a preheated oven, 325°F, for 2–2½ hours, basting every 45 minutes or so, until the meat is tender.

4 Meanwhile, prepare the beans. Heat the oil and cook the mustard and onion seeds over a low heat, letting them pop for a few seconds. Stir in the tomato paste, turmeric, and chili powder. Add the beans and a few tablespoons of hot water. Cover and cook for a few minutes. Stir in the chopped cilantro leaves and remove from the heat.

5 Preheat the broiler. Place the halved onions, cut sides up, in a heatproof dish, pour over the vinegar and cook under a preheated medium broiler for about 20 minutes until soft.

6 Serve with the spiced beans and broiled red onions and sprinkled with chopped cilantro leaves. Accompany with steamed green vegetables (cabbage, spinach, kale).

NUTRITION

• Carbohydrate 10 g
• Fat 14 g
• Protein 33 g
• Energy 293 kcal (1230 kJ)

Days 16 and 37

BREAKFAST	MID-MORNING SNACK	LUNCH	MID-AFTERNOON SNACK
⅔ cup pomegranate juice **Poached egg on 1 slice of rye or whole-wheat bread** OR **⅔ cup grapefruit juice** **Bowl of wholegrain cereal** Make with 2 cups wholegrain cereal and ⅔ cup skim or soy milk.	**1 peach or 3 plums**	**Griddled eggplants with chili toasts** (see recipe) OR **Avocado open sandwich** Make with 1 slice of wholegrain bread, topped with sliced avocado and tomato, seasoned with pepper and drizzled with a little olive oil. **Nectarine or peach and ⅔ cup lowfat fruit yogurt per person**	**Small handful of nuts and seeds** Choose from Brazil nuts, pine nuts, almonds, sunflower seeds, and pumpkin seeds.

TIP OF THE DAY

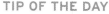

Three or more daily servings of wholegrains can reduce your risk of heart disease, certain cancers, and Type 2 diabetes by up to 30 percent.

DINNER

Cod and roasted vegetables

Place 5 oz cod and 2 oz total sliced green sweet pepper, zucchini, fennel, fresh ginger root, garlic, artichoke, and sweet potato per person together with 1 chopped onion in a dish. Drizzle with 2 tablespoons olive oil and season with salt and pepper. Bake for 30 minutes in a preheated oven, 350°F.

OR

Tofu and roasted vegetables

Prepare and cook exactly as above, substituting the cod with tofu.

Baked apples

Sprinkle 1 cooking apple per person with 1 teaspoon brown sugar, a pinch of ground cinnamon, and a few golden raisins, add a little water and bake in a preheated oven, 325°F, for about 1 hour, basting the apple skin until it turns golden brown.

Griddled Eggplants with Chili Toasts

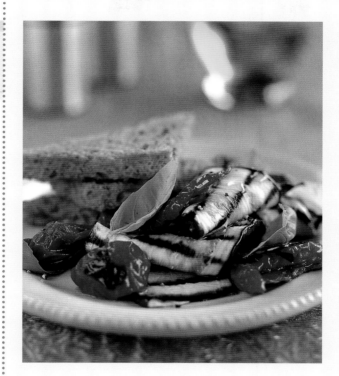

Preparation time:
15 minutes
Cooking time: 10 minutes
Serves 4

2 eggplants, about 1 lb 2 oz
in total
2 teaspoons olive oil
20 sun-dried tomatoes
2 garlic cloves, crushed
4 tablespoons lemon juice

Chili toasts
4 slices multigrain bread
1 tablespoon chili-infused oil

To garnish
4 basil leaves
pepper

1 Prepare the chili toasts. Remove the crusts from each slice of bread and cut the remaining bread into 2 neat triangles. Brush each side of the bread with chili-infused oil and put the bread on an ovenproof baking sheet.

2 Cut the eggplants lengthwise into ¼ in slices and season with pepper.

3 Put the chili toasts in a preheated oven, 425°F, and cook for 8–10 minutes until they are crisp and golden.

4 Meanwhile, oil a ridged griddle pan and heat it. Put the eggplant slices and sun-dried tomatoes on the pan with the garlic and cook for about 4 minutes until they start to soften. Turn over the eggplants and cook for an additional 4 minutes. Finally, add the lemon juice.

5 Remove the chili toasts from the oven and serve with the eggplant and tomato piled high in the center of each plate and garnished with basil leaves and pepper.

NUTRITION

- Carbohydrate 15 g
- Fat 6 g
- Protein 4 g
- Energy 122 kcal (513 kJ)

Days 17 and 38

BREAKFAST

Fruit smoothie
Blend ½ mango and 1
banana with ⅔ cup skim or
soy milk and 6 tablespoons
apple juice, then sprinkle
with a few pumpkin seeds.

OR

⅔ cup apple juice

Bowl of porridge
Make with ¾ cup rolled
oats and ¾ cup skim or soy
milk, and top with a few
blueberries.

MID-MORNING SNACK

**Small handful of white
grapes or an apple**

LUNCH

**½ 13 oz can vegetable
soup and 1 slice of
wholegrain or rye bread**

OR

**Cottage cheese and
herb sandwich**
Sandwich 2 slices rye or
whole-wheat bread with
⅓ cup cottage cheese and
some chopped scallions
and fresh herbs (cilantro,
parsley, chives).

Apple

MID-AFTERNOON SNACK

**2 oatcakes topped with
1 teaspoon hummus**

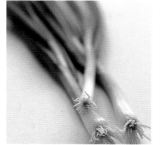

TIP OF THE DAY

Are you hungry? Think
about this really hard
before you find yourself
reaching for a snack:
perhaps a glass of water
would help, or call a
friend for a chat.

DINNER

Spiced chicken and pearl barley
(see recipe)

OR

Vegetarian chili
Serves 4

Sauté 1 chopped onion, 3 crushed garlic cloves, and ½ teaspoon chili powder in 2 tablespoons vegetable stock. Add 1 tablespoon each tomato paste and paprika and cook for 1 minute. Add a drained 13 oz can each red kidney beans and lima beans and 1 lb total sliced carrots, zucchini, sweet peppers, mushrooms, and cauliflower. Simmer until the vegetables are soft. Serve with 1 whole-wheat pita per person.

Fresh pineapple
Use 1 large slice (about 5 oz) per person.

Spiced Chicken and Pearl Barley

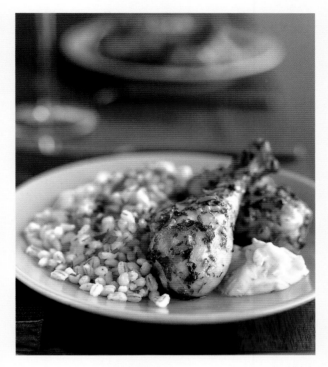

1 Combine all the ingredients for the spice mix in a bowl. Rub the spice mix all over the chicken flesh. Set the chicken aside for at least 2 hours to absorb the flavors.

2 Prepare the pearl barley. Heat the oil in a large, heavy skillet and cook the onion gently until soft, stirring so it does not brown. Add the washed barley and cook for 2 minutes. Pour in the stock and simmer for 1 hour, stirring occasionally, until all the fluid has been absorbed and the grains are soft.

3 Meanwhile, cook the chicken, uncovered, in a preheated oven, 375°F, for 30–40 minutes until it is tender throughout.

4 Make the raita. Combine the yogurt and grated cucumber and sprinkle some cumin on the top.

5 When the chicken and pearl barley are cooked, garnish the chicken with chopped parsley and serve immediately with the pearl barley and raita. Accompany with mixed salad leaves (chicory, arugula, lamb's lettuce).

Preparation time:
45 minutes, plus marinating
Cooking time: 1 hour
Serves 4

2 lb chicken pieces on the bone, skin removed
chopped parsley, to garnish

Spice mix
1 large onion, finely chopped
2 garlic cloves, chopped
½ teaspoon ground cumin
¼ teaspoon paprika
¼–½ teaspoon crushed dried chilies
1–2 pinches saffron threads
6 tablespoons finely chopped cilantro
6 tablespoons finely chopped flat-leaf parsley
2 tablespoons olive oil
2 tablespoons lemon juice

Pearl barley
1 teaspoon vegetable oil
1 small onion, chopped
1 cup pearl barley
3¾ cups chicken stock

Raita
⅔ cup lowfat plain yogurt
4 oz cucumber, grated
pinch of ground cumin

NUTRITION

- Carbohydrate 52 g
- Fat 13 g
- Protein 30 g
- Energy 428 kcal (1800 kJ)

Days 18 and 39

BREAKFAST

Small glass of tomato juice

Bowl of granola
Make with 1 cup sugar-free granola and ⅔ cup skim or soy milk, topped with a small handful of raspberries.

OR

⅔ cup pineapple juice

Ham and mushroom omelet
Make with 2 eggs, a few mushrooms and 1 oz chopped lean ham.

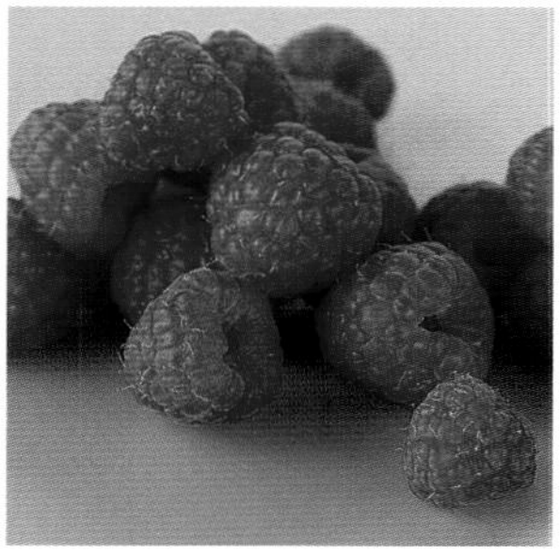

MID-MORNING SNACK

Apple or banana

LUNCH

Spicy vegetable roast
(see recipe)

OR

Cottage cheese and salad
Season ½ cup cottage cheese with paprika and serve with mixed salad leaves (arugula, baby spinach, radicchio), topped with 6 cherry tomatoes and dressed with 1 teaspoon olive oil mixed with lemon juice.

MID-AFTERNOON SNACK

2 rice cakes spread thinly with peanut butter

TIP OF THE DAY

Berries are packed with fiber, so they will keep you feeling fuller for longer. They also contain powerful cancer-fighting antioxidants.

DINNER

Ginger baked chicken
Serves 4

Marinate 4 skinless chicken breasts (5 oz each) overnight in ½ in grated fresh ginger root, 1 crushed garlic clove, 2 chopped lemon slices, 3 tablespoons soy sauce, and 4 tablespoons unsweetened apple juice. Cover with foil and bake in a preheated oven, 400°F, for 30–40 minutes. Serve with spinach and boiled new potatoes.

OR

Tofu with vegetables
Serves 4

Sprinkle 12 oz zucchini and 8 oz eggplant, cut into chunks, 8 oz halved tomatoes, 1 red sweet pepper, 1 yellow sweet pepper, and 1 onion, all quartered, and 6 cloves garlic with 5 tablespoons olive oil and salt and pepper. Roast in a preheated oven, 400°F, for 45 minutes. Serve with 4 oz baked tofu per person.

Apple or pear per person

Spicy Vegetable Roast

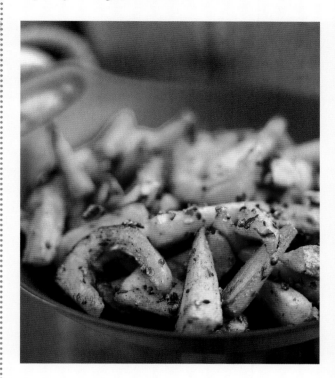

**Preparation time:
15 minutes
Cooking time:
35–40 minutes
Serves 6**

1 teaspoon fennel seeds
1 teaspoon cumin seeds
1 teaspoon coriander seeds
½ teaspoon turmeric
½ teaspoon paprika
2 garlic cloves, chopped
3 tablespoons olive oil
1 lb butternut squash,
   peeled, halved, seeded, and
   thickly sliced
4 small parsnips, about
   14 oz in total, cut into
   quarters
3 carrots, about 10 oz in
   total, cut into thick strips
salt and pepper

1 Crush the seeds using a mortar and pestle or use the end of a rolling pin. Transfer to a large plastic bag and add the turmeric, paprika, garlic, oil, and salt and pepper. Squeeze the bag to mix the contents together.

2 Add the vegetables to the plastic bag, grip the top edge to seal and toss together until the vegetables are coated with the spices.

3 Tip the vegetables into a roasting pan and bake in a preheated oven, 400°F, for 35–40 minutes, turning once until browned and tender. Transfer to a serving dish.

NUTRITION

• Carbohydrate 20 g
• Fat 7 g
• Protein 3 g
• Energy 147 kcal (619 kJ)

Days 19 and 40

BREAKFAST

Small glass of pomegranate juice

Bowl of porridge
Make with ¾ cup rolled oats and ¾ cup skim or soy milk.

OR

⅔ cup apple juice

Poached egg on 1 slice of wholegrain bread

MID-MORNING SNACK

Orange or pear

LUNCH

Avocado and sunflower seed salad
Arrange avocado slices and a sprinkling of sunflower seeds on mixed salad leaves (radicchio, lamb's lettuce, watercress) with 6 cherry tomatoes and sliced cucumber. Drizzle with a dressing of 1 teaspoon each olive oil, white wine vinegar, and lemon juice per person.

OR

Shrimp tortilla
Fill a flour tortilla with 3 oz shrimp (or chicken), chopped tomatoes, cucumber, and red sweet pepper, mixed with 2 tablespoons lowfat plain yogurt, a squeeze of lemon juice, and chopped chili (optional). (Substitute the flour tortilla with 2 slices of wholegrain bread if preferred.)

Small bowl of strawberries

MID-AFTERNOON SNACK

Small handful of mixed nuts
Choose from walnuts, almonds, Brazil nuts, or pine nuts.

TIP OF THE DAY

If you are working, prepare your lunch the night before and take it with you.

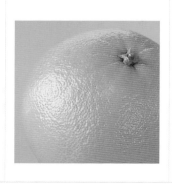

DINNER

Angler fish with asparagus
Serves 4

Mix 2 crushed garlic cloves, 1 teaspoon shredded fresh ginger root, 2 tablespoons soy sauce, and ¼ teaspoon rice vinegar, and pour over 1¼ lb boned, cubed angler fish tail. Cover the dish. Drizzle 7 oz asparagus with olive oil. Roast fish and asparagus in a preheated oven, 400°F, for 15–20 minutes. Serve with a leafy green vegetable.

OR

Bean and feta stir-fry
Serves 4

Fry 2–3 chopped garlic cloves and 1 chopped onion in 1 tablespoon olive oil. Add 3 chopped tomatoes, a drained 13 oz can each red kidney and flageolet beans, 3 tablespoons black olives, and 1 tablespoon soy sauce and lemon juice. Cook for 4–5 minutes. Add 4 oz feta cheese and season with fresh herbs and pepper.

Almondy angel cakes
(see recipe)

Almondy Angel Cakes

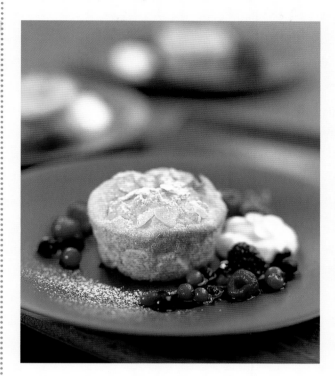

**Preparation time:
15 minutes**

Serves 6

**4 egg whites
1½ tablespoons superfine
  sugar
½ cup ground almonds
generous pinch of cream
  of tartar
2 tablespoons slivered
  almonds
13 oz frozen mixed berry
  fruits
¾ cup lowfat plain yogurt**

1 Lightly oil 6 sections of a deep muffin pan and line the bases with circles of waxed paper.

2 Beat the egg whites until stiff, moist peaks form. Beat in the sugar, a teaspoonful at a time, until it has all been added and continue to beat for a minute or two until the mixture is thick and glossy.

3 Fold in the ground almonds and cream of tartar and spoon the mixture into the sections of the muffin pan. Sprinkle the slivered almonds over the tops.

4 Cook in a preheated oven, 350°F, for 10–12 minutes until golden brown and set. Loosen the edges of the cakes with a knife and lift them onto a cooling rack.

5 Warm the fruits in a saucepan. Arrange the angel cakes on serving plates, add a spoonful of yogurt to each, and spoon the fruits around.

NUTRITION

- Carbohydrate 8 g
- Fat 9 g
- Protein 7 g
- Energy 140 kcal (583 kJ)

Days 20 and 41

BREAKFAST

²⁄₃ cup apple and mango juice

2 large broiled tomatoes on 1 slice of wholegrain toast spread thinly with olive oil spread

OR

¾ cup pomegranate juice

Crunchy yogurt
Mix 1 tablespoon each toasted jumbo oats and mixed berries (strawberries, blueberries, blackberries, and raspberries) into ²⁄₃ cup lowfat plain yogurt and sprinkle sesame and sunflower seeds on top.

MID-MORNING SNACK

Peach or nectarine and 3 fresh or dried apricots

LUNCH

Hot chicken liver salad (see recipe)

OR

Rice salad
Serves 4

Mix together juice of 1 lemon, 1 crushed garlic clove, 1 tablespoon olive oil, and salt and pepper. Stir the following into ¼ cup each cooked brown rice and cooked millet: 1 chopped bunch scallions, 2 diced sweet peppers, 2 chopped large tomatoes, ½ chopped cucumber, ½ cup chopped mixed nuts (walnuts, almonds, Brazil nuts). Then pour the dressing over the salad and leave in the refrigerator to chill.

MID-AFTERNOON SNACK

2 rice cakes, spread thinly with tahini or topped with 2 tablespoons cottage cheese

TIP OF THE DAY

Oats are complex carbohydrates that release energy slowly, so you feel fuller for longer. They also help to stabilize blood sugar, discouraging you from snacking.

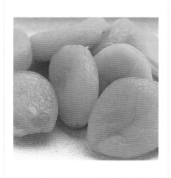

DINNER

Baked trout
Serves 4

Sprinkle 1 trout fillet (1¼ lb) with chopped dill and scallions, lemon pepper and salt. Cover with foil and bake in a preheated oven, 400°F, for 15–20 minutes. Garnish with toasted pine nuts and orange slices and serve with zucchini, spinach, and carrots.

OR

Vegetable penne
Serves 4

Fry 1 chopped onion and 1 chopped garlic clove in 2 tablespoons olive oil until soft. Add a 7 oz can tomatoes, 1 tablespoon each tomato paste and lemon juice, and salt and pepper. Simmer for 10–15 minutes. Stir in 4 oz each torn spinach and sliced zucchini, 2 oz baby corn, 2 tablespoons fresh herbs. Simmer for 2 minutes. Serve with 12 oz whole-wheat pasta.

Baked bananas
(see recipe on page 39)

Hot Chicken Liver Salad

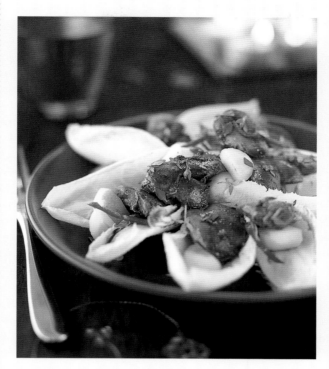

Preparation time:
5 minutes, plus soaking
Cooking time: 5 minutes
Serves 4

13 oz chicken livers,
  trimmed and halved
¼ cup milk
2 teaspoons chopped thyme
1 tablespoon olive oil
2 garlic cloves, crushed
1 red chili pepper, sliced
  thinly (optional)
7 oz can water chestnuts,
  drained and halved

To serve
7 oz Belgian endive, leaves
  separated
1½–2 tablespoons balsamic
  vinegar

1 Soak the liver in milk for 30 minutes to remove any bitterness. Discard the milk and pat the liver dry with paper towels. Sprinkle the thyme over both sides of the liver.

2 Heat the oil in a large skillet and add the garlic and sliced chili (if using). Allow the garlic and chili to soften for 30 seconds, then add the chicken livers and water chestnuts.

3 Cook over a medium heat for 3–4 minutes, until the liver is browned on the outside but still pink in the middle.

4 Serve on a bed of crispy raw Belgian endive, drizzled with balsamic vinegar and any remaining pan juices.

NUTRITION

- Carbohydrate 9 g
- Fat 10 g
- Protein 21 g
- Energy 199 kcal (835 kJ)

Days 21 and 42

BREAKFAST

Banana smoothie
Blend together 1 banana, ⅔ cup skim milk and ⅔ cup lowfat plain yogurt, then sprinkle with sunflower seeds.

OR

⅔ cup orange juice

Bowl of porridge
Make with ½ cup millet or ¾ cup rolled oats and ¾ cup skim or soy milk, sprinkled with flax seeds.

MID-MORNING SNACK

Apple or pear

LUNCH

Savory omelet
Make with 2 eggs, chopped mushrooms, red sweet pepper and onion, and serve with mixed salad leaves (watercress, arugula, lamb's lettuce).

OR

Tuna salad
Drain a 6½ oz can tuna and mix with 1 teaspoon olive oil and juice of ½ lemon, chopped scallions and chives. Serve the tuna on a bed of mixed salad leaves (chicory, lettuce, baby spinach) with 6 cherry tomatoes.

MID-AFTERNOON SNACK

Handful of grapes or 2 plums

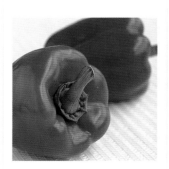

TIP OF THE DAY

The spice in peppers—capsaicin—speeds up your metabolism, helping you to burn fat.

DINNER

Flounder parcels
(see recipe)

OR

Steak and mixed rice

Fry 1 chopped onion in 1 tablespoon olive oil until brown. Add 1 cup wild rice and 2 cups vegetable stock and simmer until the stock has been absorbed. Meanwhile, broil 5 oz steak per person. Serve with the rice and steamed vegetables.

Mango sorbet
Serves 6

Boil ¼ cup light cane sugar in ¾ cup water until dissolved, then cool. Stir in the pureed flesh of 1 mango and juice of 1 lb clementines and freeze in a plastic box for 2–3 hours until semifrozen. Beat well, then freeze and beat again. Mix in 1 egg white and freeze until solid. Slice 1 mango and toss in the grated zest and juice of 1 lime. Soften the sorbet at room temperature for 15 minutes and serve with the mango slices.

Flounder Parcels

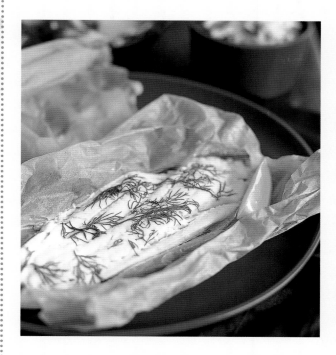

Preparation time:
30 minutes
Cooking time: 10 minutes
Serves 4

1 fennel bulb, about 12 oz
2 red chilies, seeded and
   chopped
4 tablespoons lemon juice
2 teaspoons olive oil
4 flounder fillets, about
   1 lb 6 oz in total
1 small handful chopped dill
½ lemon, cut into wedges,
   to garnish

Radicchio and orange salad
7 oz red radicchio leaves
2 large oranges, peeled and
   pith removed, separated
   into segments

1 Finely chop the fennel bulb and put it in a bowl with the chopped chilies. Add the lemon juice and olive oil to the fennel and set aside.

2 Cut 4 sheets of parchment paper, each 14 x 7 in, and fold them in half widthwise. Lay ½ sheet over a plate and arrange a fish fillet on one side of the fold. Sprinkle over some chopped dill and fold over the paper to enclose the filling. Fold in the edges and pleat to secure. Repeat with the remaining fish.

3 Place the wrapped fish on a baking sheet and cook in a preheated oven, 425°F, for about 8 minutes or until the paper is puffed up and brown.

4 Make the salad by combining the radicchio with the orange segments.

5 Place each fish parcel on a large plate and cut an X-shaped slit in the top and curl back the paper, or pull the paper apart to open the parcel, releasing a fragrant puff of steam. Serve with individual side bowls of the fennel and chili mixture and radicchio and orange salad, and garnish with a lemon wedge.

NUTRITION

- Carbohydrate 13 g
- Fat 6 g
- Protein 32 g
- Energy 234 kcal (988 kJ)

THE WAISTLINE

1   2   3   4   5   6   7   8   9   10   11   12   13

EXERCISE PLAN

14 | 15 | 16 | 17 | 18 | 19 | 20 | 21 | 22 | 23 | 24 | 25 | 26

HOW THE EXERCISE PLAN WORKS

The Waistline Diet Plan will enable you to lose weight and feel healthier and more energized. At the same time, you can tone and flatten your stomach, and sculpt your hips, thighs, and buttocks, by following the Waistline Exercise Plan. The combination of toning workouts and aerobic exercise will not only give you a new shape, it will also help you to achieve a new sense of confidence and wellbeing.

WHAT WILL IT DO FOR ME?

Exercise brings so many different benefits. Not only does it make you healthier and less stressed, it also makes you look and feel great and it even helps you to lose weight by speeding up your metabolism and enabling your body to burn fat for longer. Some people worry that they are too busy to commit to regular exercise or even that they are too unfit to begin. The Waistline Exercise Plan is all about showing how easy it is to bring regular exercise into your life, with short but effective sessions that can be fitted into your daily schedule without taking up too much of your time.

The Waistline Exercise Plan works by combining specific toning exercises that focus on the muscles of the stomach, hips, thighs, and buttocks with an aerobic "interval" exercise session that targets your heart and lungs, helping you to build strength and stamina and burn fat. It is this combination of aerobic and toning exercise that will help you to achieve a flatter, thinner you, which is why you must incorporate both sets of activities into your Plan—so don't forget to do one weekly aerobic session at the very least.

WHO IS IT FOR?

This exercise regime is suitable for everyone, from absolute beginners to those who exercise regularly. The Waistline Exercise Plan can be adapted to take into account your own specific exercise needs, so long as you achieve the minimum level of toning and exercise activity. Once you begin to exercise you will soon see the benefits. The more you exercise, the more energy you will have and the more you will want to exercise.

Continuing to use the Waistline Exercise Plan on a regular basis will mean you can maintain a healthy body-fat level in the future.

HOW MUCH SHOULD I DO?

To get real benefit from the Waistline Exercise Plan, you should do the toning exercises for 10 minutes per session (excluding warm-up and cool-down exercises), 3 times a day, 5 times a week. Along with these, you also need to include a 20-minute aerobic session each week. If you find this too much at first, begin with just 10 minutes of exercises per day, 5 days a week, along with your 20-minute aerobic session—but bear in mind that the results will be slower. You can then increase the duration and frequency of your exercise and aerobic sessions, building up to 30 minutes total of toning exercises, 5 days a week and 2 or more aerobic sessions. You must have 2 rest days per week, but that doesn't rule out a brisk walk or short swim on these days.

AEROBIC EXERCISES

- Brisk walking
- Jogging
- Skipping
- Step
- Dancing
- Swimming
- Cycling
- Rowing
- Basketball
- Tennis
- Squash
- Hockey
- Basketball
- Rollerblading

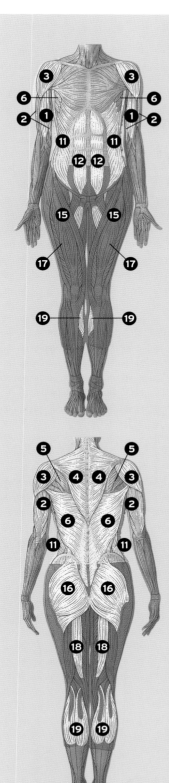

IMPORTANT MUSCLES

1 **Biceps**—front of the upper arm, used to move the arm.

2 **Triceps**—back of the upper arm, used to move the arm.

3 **Deltoid**—encloses the shoulder and upper arm, used to move the arm backward and forward.

4 **Trapezius**—runs down the back of the neck and along the shoulders, used to extend the head.

5 **Rhomboid**—attaches the shoulder blades to the spine. Mostly lies beneath the trapezius muscle.

6 **Latissimus dorsi**—popularly referred to as "lats," it runs from the lower chest into the lumbar region. It pulls the shoulders down and back and the body upward.

7 **Erector spinae**—(not shown) found at the back of the neck, chest, and abdomen. This important muscle extends the spine and holds the body upright.

8 **Quadratus lumborum**—(not shown) deep interior waist muscle. It bends the torso sideways.

9 **Transversus abdominis**—(not shown) deep internal muscle that runs across the abdomen. It applies pressure to the abdomen and holds the organs in place. It lies beneath the internal oblique muscle (see 10).

10 **Internal oblique**—(not shown) horizontally crosses the abdomen, compresses the abdomen, and moves the trunk. It lies beneath the external oblique muscle (see 11).

11 **External oblique**—side muscle of the abdomen. It compresses the abdomen and is used when moving the trunk in any direction.

12 **Rectus abdominis**—popularly known as the "abs," this muscle runs vertically down the entire front of the abdomen. This postural muscle draws the front of the pelvis upward.

13 **Perineum**—(not shown) an internal muscle. It forms the pelvic floor and attaches to the pelvic wall, which is located deep in the pelvic cavity.

14 **Psoas**—(not shown) this deep muscle is part of the hip flexor. It runs from the front of the femur to the lumbar region of the spine. It acts to bring the thigh forward at the hip.

15 **Adductor**—an inner thigh muscle, used for moving the leg inward.

16 **Gluteus maximus**—forms the buttocks. It is used for walking, running, and jumping.

17 **Quadriceps extensor**—runs down the middle of the front of the thigh. It performs the opposite movement to the semitendinosus or hamstrings.

18 **Semitendinosus**—also known as the hamstrings. This muscle runs down the middle of the back of the thigh. Used to extend the thigh and to flex the leg at the knee joint.

19 **Gastrocnemius**—this muscle runs down the back of the lower leg and forms the greater part of the calf. It gives the force when walking and running.

20 MINUTES OF AEROBIC EXERCISE

Aerobic exercise requires the use of oxygen and involves the lungs, heart, and blood circulation system of the body. It helps to burn calories, reduces stress levels and the production of cortisol, lowers blood pressure, develops cardiovascular fitness, and improves your cholesterol levels. Once you find your session easy, or you wish to lose weight more quickly, you can build more sessions into your week.

During your 20-minute "interval" exercise session, you should alternate bouts of short, sharp, intense activity with short periods of lower intensity activity. This method of exercising has been shown to promote weight loss. For example, if you are jogging you would warm up for 5 minutes, then run hard and fast for 1–2 minutes (depending on your fitness level), then jog to

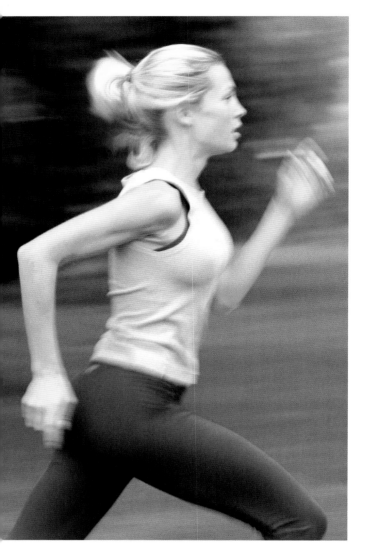

recover for another 2 minutes. You would then simply repeat the process for 20 minutes. This method can be applied to all the aerobic exercise suggestions (see panel on page 72).

If you find it difficult to exercise for the full 20 minutes to begin with, gradually build yourself up to it. You can choose a mix of several aerobic exercises if you prefer: for example, running and rowing, or cycling, stepping, and dancing. To avoid stiffness or injury, make sure you remember both to warm up and cool down thoroughly both before and after any aerobic session (see below).

PUTTING IT ALL TOGETHER

Before you begin an exercise session, you need to make sure your muscles are thoroughly warmed up. Try brisk walking, jogging on the spot, gentle or stationary cycling, rowing, stepping, or skipping for around 5 minutes. You should feel warm but not exhausted.

- Move on to the warm-up stretches on pages 77–83. These are important, so do not miss them out.
- Now select at least 3 exercises from pages 84–95 (for the buttocks, hips, and thighs) and 5 from pages 96–117 (for the stomach).
- Follow these with the cool-down stretches on pages 118–123. To cool down, you can also use some of the warm-up stretches on pages 77–83.

Reps and sets

Each exercise specifies the number of reps (repetitions) and sets you should perform. Reps are the number of times you repeat an exercise in one go, while a set is the completed number of repetitions. So, if you perform 3 sets of 8 reps each, you will perform 24 repetitions of the exercise in all.

For exercises performed on both sides of the body, the number of reps specified is for one side only.

USING HAND WEIGHTS

When you start to feel fitter and stronger, use small hand weights to increase the resistance training effect of the following exercises:

- **Knee lifts** (see page 83)
- **Squats** (see page 84)
- **Arabesque** (see page 90)
- **Lunges with lateral raises** (see page 92)

Work those muscles!

At the start of each exercise, you will be told which muscles are being targeted. Unless you already know which muscles are which, you will probably find it useful to refer to the diagrams and explanations on page 73, which describe where the important muscles in the body are and what they do.

SAMPLE WORKOUT ROUTINE

Warm-up
- Upper body warm-up (see page 77)
- Side stretch (see page 78)
- Side twist (see page 79)
- Calf stretch (see page 80)
- Hamstring stretch (see page 81)
- Quads stretch (see page 82)
- Knee lifts (see page 83)

Toning exercises
- Squats (see page 84)
- Buttock kicks (see page 86)
- Bottom lifts (see page 87)
- Leg lifts (see page 88)
- Lunges with lateral raises (see page 92)
- Inner thigh lifts (see page 94)
- Roll-ups (see page 96)
- Scissors (see page 102)
- The plank (see page 104)
- Tummy tighteners (see page 108)
- Oblique crunch (see page 110)

Cool-down
- Groin stretch (see page 118)
- Inner thigh stretch (see page 119)
- Spinal twist (see page 120)
- Pose of the child (see page 122)

COMFORT AND SAFETY

Wear appropriate clothing for your workout. Anything comfortable such as a T-shirt and leggings or shorts is fine, and for women a sports bra is a good investment. You will need a suitable pair of trainers to act as shock absorbers and protect your feet. A towel or floor mat will also be useful to help protect your knees, hips, and back.

It is important that you do not become dehydrated: drink water before, during, and after exercise. Water keeps your body hydrated, flushes out toxins, repairs cells, and helps to keep your skin looking good. Mineral or filtered water is best.

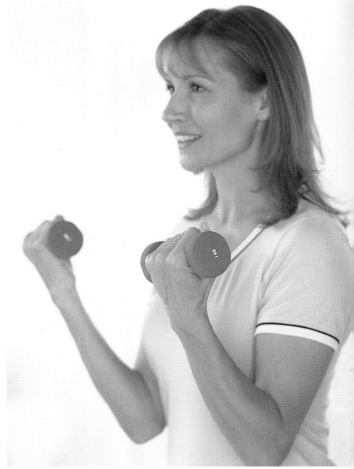

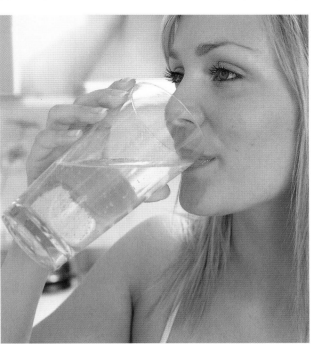

Steps

Before you begin exercising, warm up the body with some gentle aerobic exercise, such as jogging on the spot, skipping, or stepping, then follow with some of the warm-up stretches on pages 77–83.

· REPS 5–10 MINS

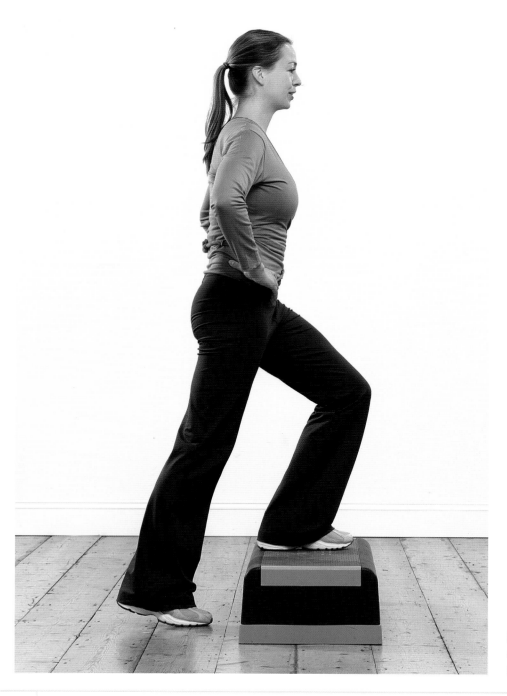

Step on and off a step alternately with each foot.

Upper body warm-up

| • REPS 10 |
| • SETS 1–2 |

These upper body warm-up exercises are good for opening the chest, stretching the pectoral muscles, and lengthening the spine.

WATCHPOINTS

• As you circle, keep your back long and straight and your shoulders down

• Stretch your arms and fingers straight up, palms facing in

• Keep your stomach pulled in

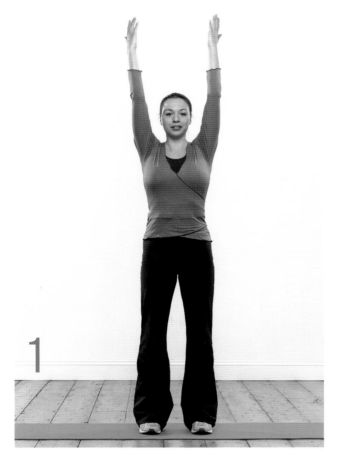

1

Stand with your feet facing forward and hip-width apart, your stomach pulled in, and your arms hanging loosely at your sides. Circle your arms forward and around. Repeat in a backward circular motion.

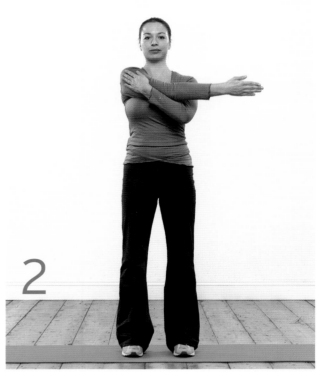

2

Cross your right arm in front of your body. Place your left hand on your right upper arm and press firmly. Hold for a count of 10, then repeat with your other arm.

Side stretch

- REPS 5–8
- SETS 1

This exercise will stretch and tone the external oblique muscles that run down the sides of your waist. You will soon find that your hand can reach down past your knee.

WATCHPOINTS

- Try to keep your stomach pulled in

- Breathe out on the way down and in on the way up

- Allow your head to drop right over to your shoulder as you stretch

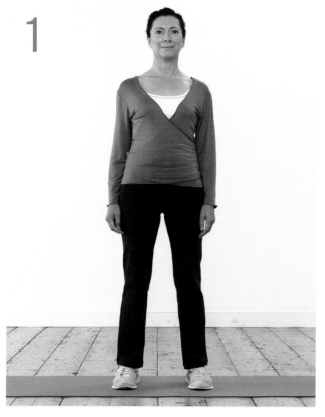

1

Stand with your feet facing forward and hip-width apart, with your arms hanging loosely at your sides.

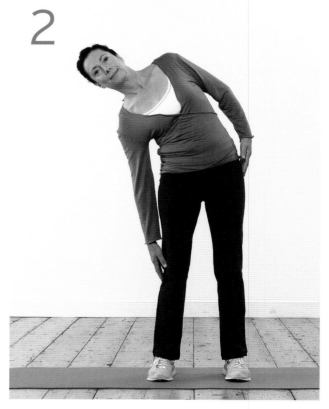

2

Exhale and slide your right arm down your right side, letting your shoulders and head drop to the right, and stretching your fingers downward. Make sure you pull in your stomach to maximize the stretch. Inhale and return to the starting position. Repeat on the left side.

Side twist

• **REPS 10**
• **SETS 1**

This is a great exercise for toning and tightening your waist, working on the external oblique muscles.

WATCHPOINTS

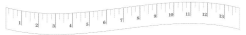

• **Make sure your knees are slightly bent**

• **Remember to push your elbows back**

• **Keep your back long**

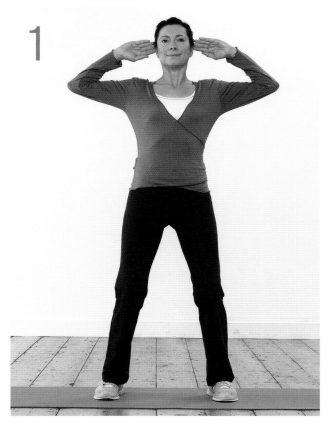

1

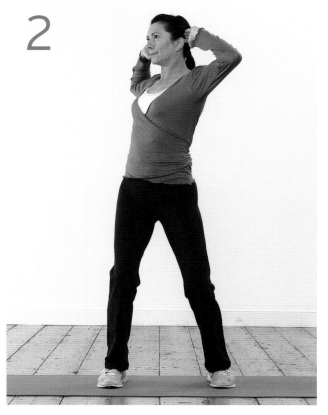

2

Stand with your feet facing forward and slightly wider than hip-width apart. Place your hands each side of your head, elbows facing outward. Bend your knees slightly.

Twist your body to the right, pushing both elbows backward. Return to the starting position and then repeat to the left.

Calf stretch

• **REPS 3**
• **SETS 1–5**

This movement stretches the gastrocnemius or calf muscle. It can be used for both the warm-up and the cool-down.

WATCHPOINTS

- Hold on to a bar or push against the wall to make this movement easier
- Keep your toes pointing forward

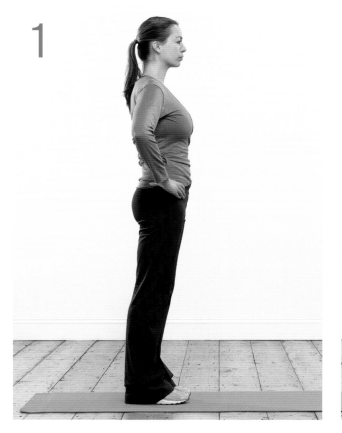

1

Stand straight, with both feet together. Put your hands on your hips and lengthen your spine.

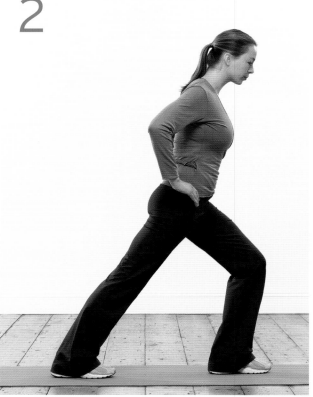

2

Step forward with your left leg. Lean from the hips, placing your weight on a slightly bent left leg. Keep your right foot straight and flat on the floor and feel the stretch through your right calf. Hold for a count of 10. Return to the starting position and repeat with your left leg.

Hamstring stretch

<table>
<tr><td>• REPS 3</td></tr>
<tr><td>• SETS 1–2</td></tr>
</table>

This stretch will lengthen the hamstrings, helping to prevent injury. It can be used for both the warm-up and the cool-down.

WATCHPOINTS

- Push out your buttocks to feel the stretch.
- Keep your chest lifted

1

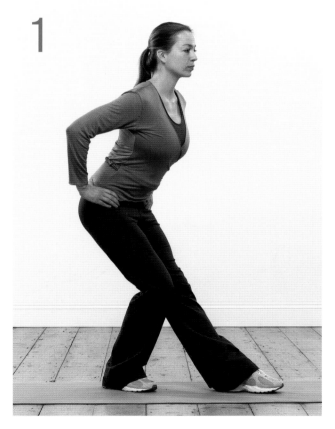

Stand with both feet together. Extend your left leg in front of you, keeping the foot on the floor. Bend your right knee. Bend from the hips and feel the stretch through the back of your left leg.

2

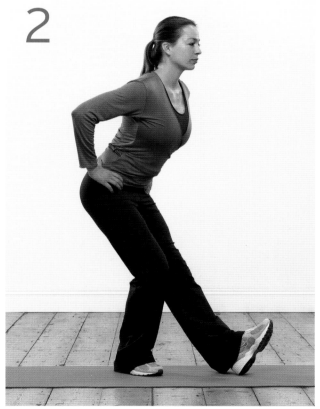

Keeping your right foot on the floor, lift the toes of your left foot toward you. Keep the heel on the floor and feel the stretch through the back of your left leg. Hold for a count of 10. Return to the starting position and repeat with your right leg.

Quads stretch

This stretch works the quadriceps muscles of the thighs. It is an excellent exercise to incorporate in both your warm-up and cool-down routines.

• **REPS 3**
• **SETS 1–2**

WATCHPOINTS

- Push your hips slightly forward to increase the stretch.

- Keep your back long and straight

- If you find it difficult to keep your balance, use a chair or wall for support

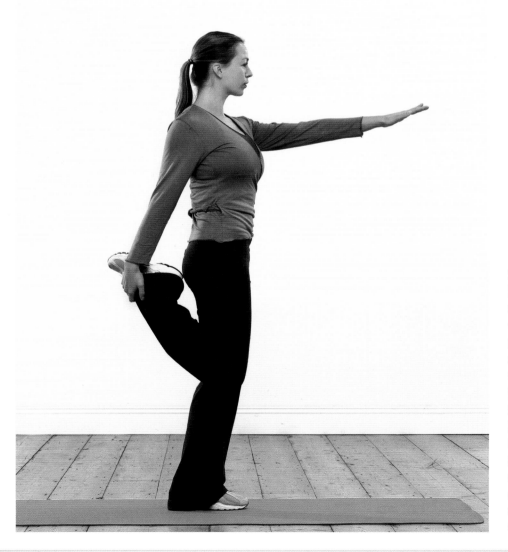

Stand with your left hand either out in front or to the side to help you balance. Bend your right knee and take hold of the front of the foot with your right hand. Pull your right heel back toward your right buttock, keeping your knees in line with each other. You will feel a stretch down the front of your thigh. Hold for a count of 10. Repeat with your left leg.

Knee lifts

This warm-up exercise is good for toning your waist as it works the stomach muscles—the external obliques and the abdominals. It also strengthens the quadriceps muscles of the thighs.

- **REPS 10–16**
- **SETS 1–2**

WATCHPOINTS

- **Keep your back straight and shoulders down**

- **Rotate around your waist in order to work the oblique muscles**

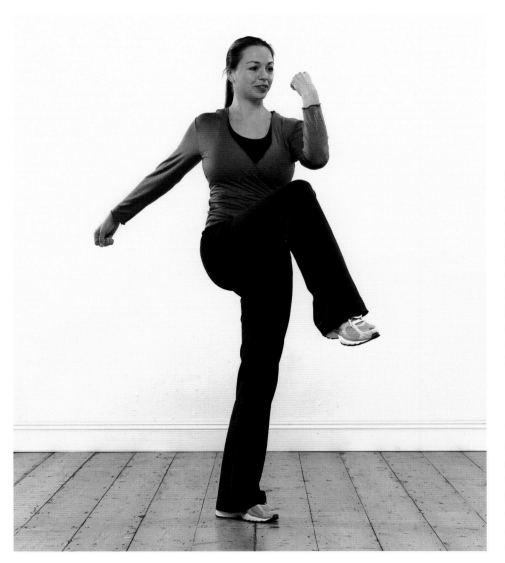

Stand with your feet facing forward and hip-width apart. Lift your right knee to chest height and take your left elbow across to your right knee. Repeat, lifting your left knee to chest height and taking your right elbow across to your left knee.

Variations

To introduce an aerobic element to this exercise, add a hop with each knee lift. To increase the intensity of the exercise, hold a hand weight in each hand.

Squats

• REPS 10
• SETS 1–3

This first exercise from the workout proper strengthens the quadriceps muscles in the thighs, the hamstrings, the gluteus medius on the hip, and the gluteus maximus in the buttocks.

WATCHPOINTS

- Keep your feet flat on the floor
- Don't squat down too quickly
- Make sure your buttocks do not go any lower than your knees

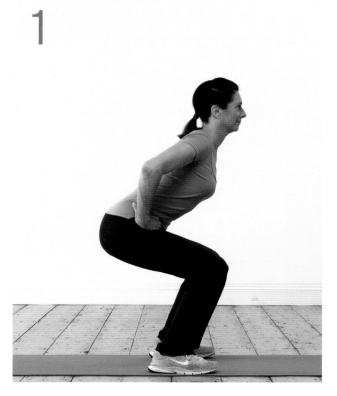

1

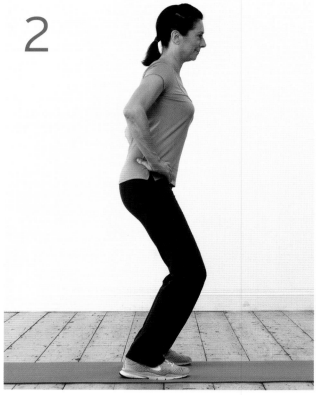

2

Stand with your feet facing forward and hip-width apart. Place your hands on your hips and pull in your stomach. Keeping your back straight, bend 90 degrees at the knees, leaning forward until your body is at 90 degrees to your thighs. Keep your feet flat on the floor. Hold for a count of 3.

Using your thigh muscles, push back up to the starting position but do not straighten your legs completely before repeating. To increase the intensity of the exercise, add hand weights.

Squat jumps

This exercise works the quadriceps, hamstrings, gluteus medius, and gluteus maximus muscles. It is more taxing than squats, and you may only manage 3 or 4 repetitions to begin with.

WATCHPOINTS

- Do only as many repetitions as you can to begin with

- Remember to bend your knees when you land

- Keep your chin and head up

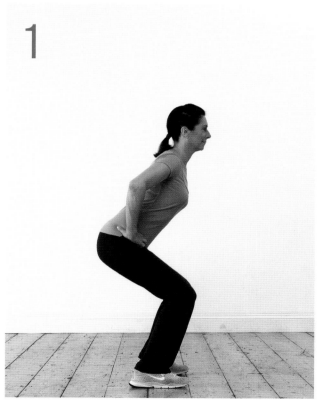

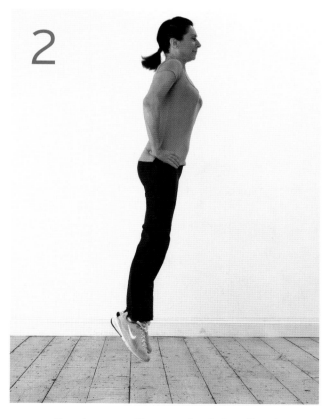

Stand with your feet facing forward and hip-width apart, your stomach pulled in, and your hands on your hips. Squat down as before.

Now jump up. Tap your heels together in mid-air and land with your feet apart, back in the squat position.

Buttock kicks

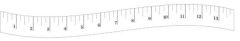

- **REPS 16**
- **SETS 1–3**

This exercise works on toning the gluteus medius and gluteus maximus muscles of your hips and buttocks, as well as the hip flexors. It also strengthens the hamstrings.

WATCHPOINTS

- Keep your stomach pulled up to your spine
- Push your leg as high as you can without strain
- Keep the exercise slow and controlled

1

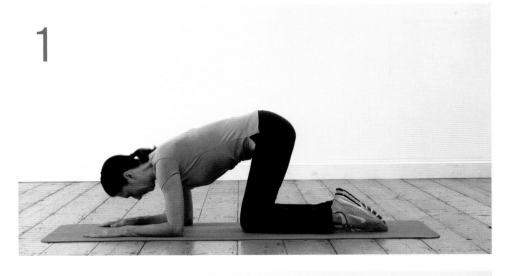

Kneel on all fours with your elbows under your chest and knees under your hips. Lower your body downward, onto your elbows.

2

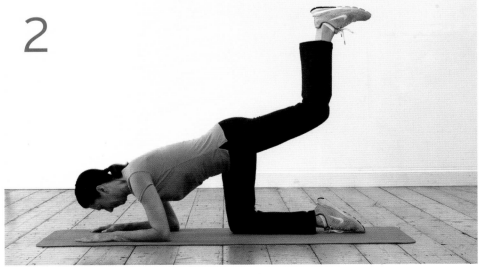

Lift your left leg off the floor, keeping your knee bent at 90 degrees, until the sole of your foot is facing the ceiling. Raise your foot high above your buttocks. Hold and squeeze your buttocks for 2 seconds. Lower your leg to the starting position and repeat with your right leg.

Bottom lifts

Strengthening the quadriceps muscles and the gluteus maximus and minimus muscles, this exercise tones your bottom. It also works the abdominal muscles and the lower back.

WATCHPOINTS

- Keep your bottom off the floor during the exercise
- Pull your stomach down and in tightly
- Curl up through your pelvis

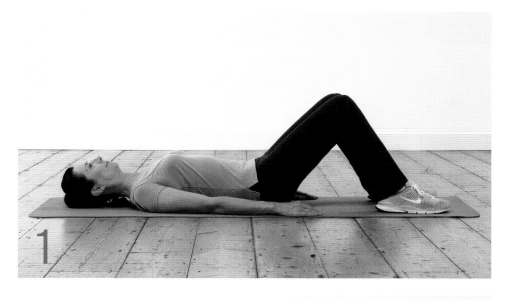

Lie on your back with both knees bent and your feet flat on the floor, hip-width apart. Place your hands flat on the floor, with your arms at the sides of your body.

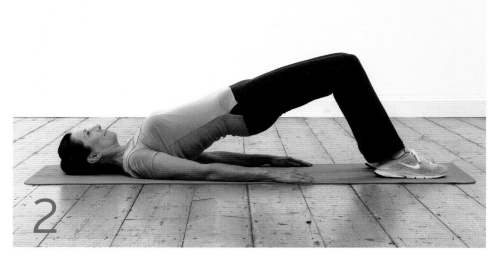

Raise your hips off the floor as far as you can. Lift and squeeze your buttocks together tightly. Hold for a count of 4, then lower your hips back down to the floor.

Leg lifts

This exercise is great for toning the legs, working the quadriceps and hamstrings. It also targets hip and buttock muscles—the gluteus maximus, minimus and medius muscles, and the hip flexor.

WATCHPOINTS

• Don't bend the knee of the lifted leg

• Keep your head down on your forearms

1

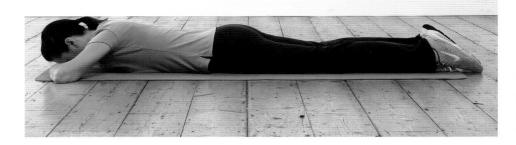

Lie face down on the floor, with your forehead resting on your forearms.

2

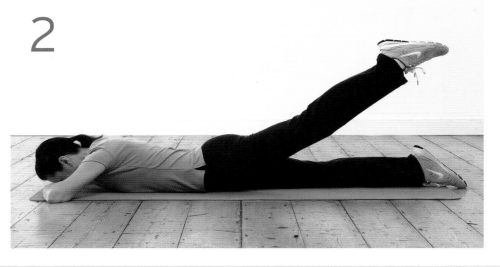

Lift up your left leg, straight out behind you. Hold for a count of 3, then lower. Repeat with your right leg.

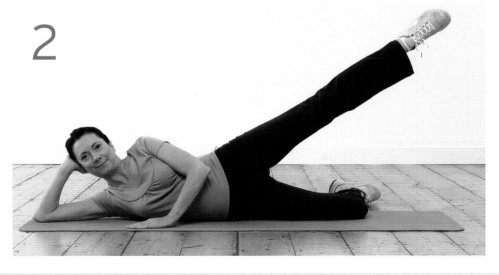

Side leg lifts

This exercise strengthens the gluteus maximus and gluteus medius muscles of the buttocks, as well as the hip flexors. You may find your legs ache to begin with, but this will ease.

> • **REPS 16**
> • **SETS 1–3**

WATCHPOINTS

- Keep your body in a straight line throughout

- To stop yourself rolling backward, push your hips forward

- Don't allow the lift to become a continuous movement—remember to hold

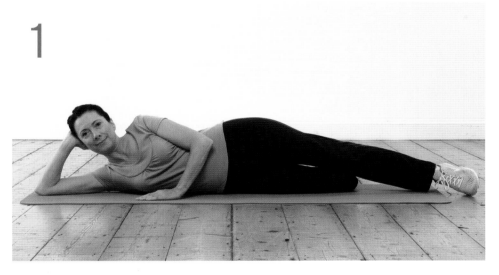

1

Lie on your right side with your body in a straight line, your right elbow bent and your right hand supporting your head. Place your left hand on the floor in front of you, close to your body, for support. Keeping your hips facing forward, bend your right knee on the floor so your right foot faces backward.

2

Lift your left leg as high as you can. Hold for a count of 2, then lower. Aim to do 16 lifts, then repeat on the other side.

Arabesque

• **REPS 16**
• **SETS 1–3**

This exercise works lower body muscles, such as the quadriceps of the thighs and the gluteus maximus muscles of the buttocks. The hip flexors and the erector spinae of the back are also targeted.

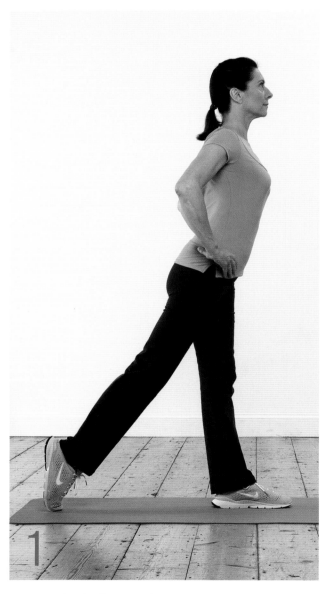

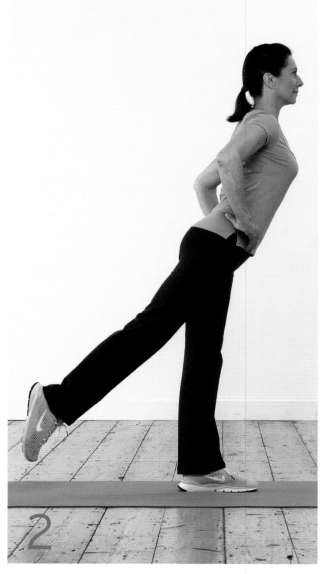

Stand with your feet together and hands on your hips. Incline your body forward slightly from the hips, keeping your back straight and head up. Stretch your right leg out straight behind you.

Lift your right leg as high as you can manage comfortably. Hold for a count of 2, then lower. Repeat with your left leg.

WATCHPOINTS

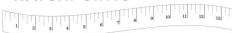

- Keep your back straight

- Make sure your hips face forward, to protect your back

- Hold on to the back of a chair if you need some support as you lift

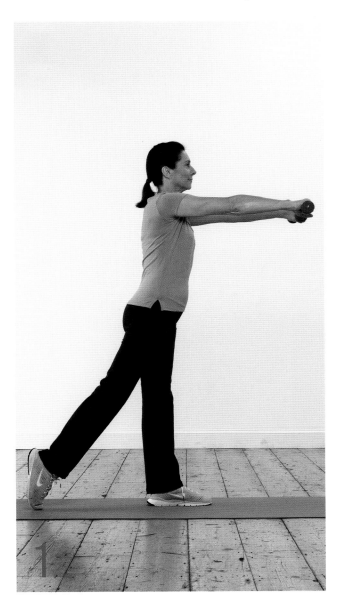

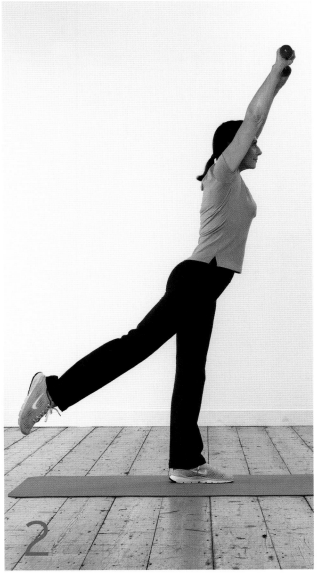

Variation

To increase the intensity of this exercise, hold a 4½ lb hand weight in each hand.

As you raise your leg, lift the hand weights straight up above your shoulder and over your head (the weights will enable you to lift your leg higher). Hold for a count of 2, then lower. Repeat with your other leg.

Lunges with lateral raises

This exercise is great for strengthening the buttocks, thighs, and calves. The gluteals, quadriceps, hamstrings, and gastrocnemius are the muscles worked here.

- **REPS 10**
- **SETS 1–3**

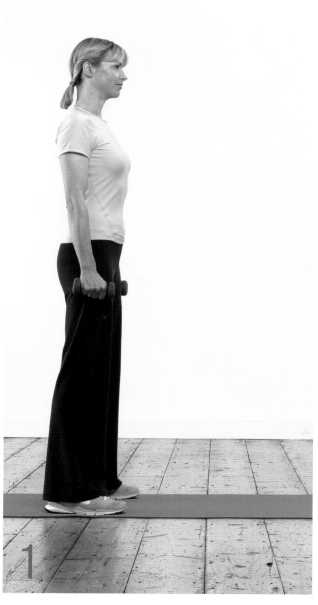

1 Stand with your feet together. Hold a light hand weight in each hand resting by your sides, palms facing in.

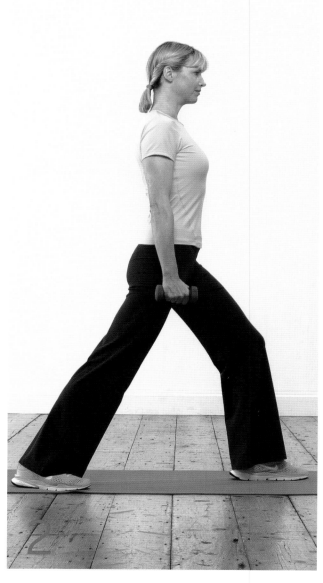

2 Take a large step forward with your left leg, keeping your stomach tight and your back straight.

WATCHPOINTS

- Don't allow your bent knee to touch the floor

- Your shoulders must be in line with your hips

- Place the weight on the heel of your front foot to work the buttock muscle

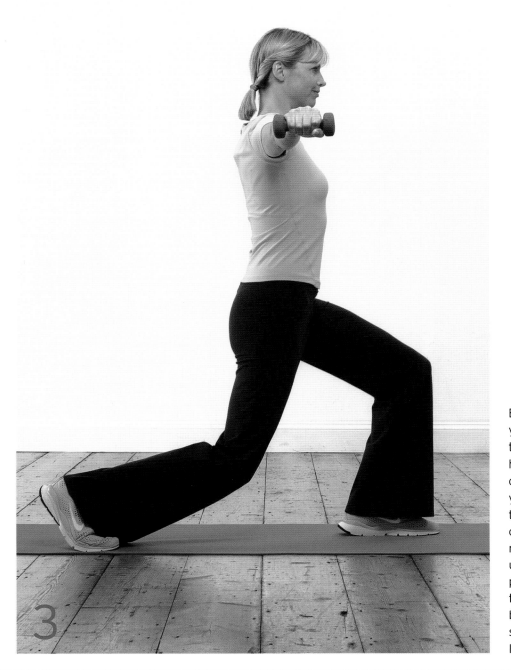

3

Bend both knees, until your right knee is close to the floor. Raise the hand weights up and out to the sides until your arms are parallel to the floor. Hold for a count of 2. Using your right thigh, push back up to the starting position. At the same time, lower your arms back down to your sides. Repeat with your left leg.

Inner thigh lifts

<table>
<tr><td>• REPS 16
• SETS 1–3</td></tr>
</table>

This exercise specifically targets the hip adductor muscles of the inner thigh. You will need to keep your inner thigh tight throughout the exercise in order to work these muscles properly.

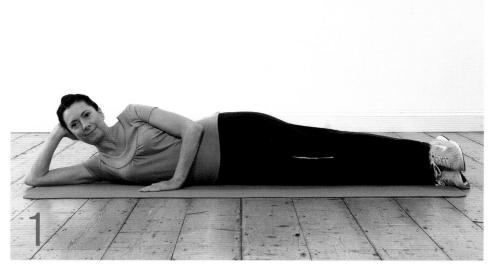

Lie on your right side with your body in a straight line, your right elbow bent, and your right hand supporting your head. Place your left hand in front of you, close to your body, for support.

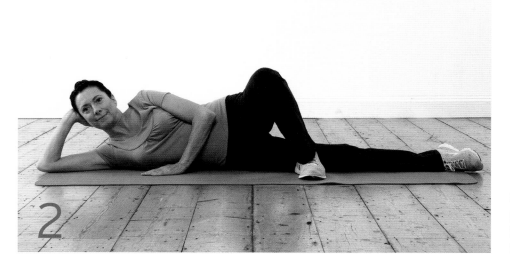

Bend your left leg and place your foot flat on the floor so that it is in front of you.

WATCHPOINTS

- Ensure this is not a continuous movement—remember to hold

- Don't let your leg touch the floor in between lifts

- To stop yourself rolling back, push your hips forward

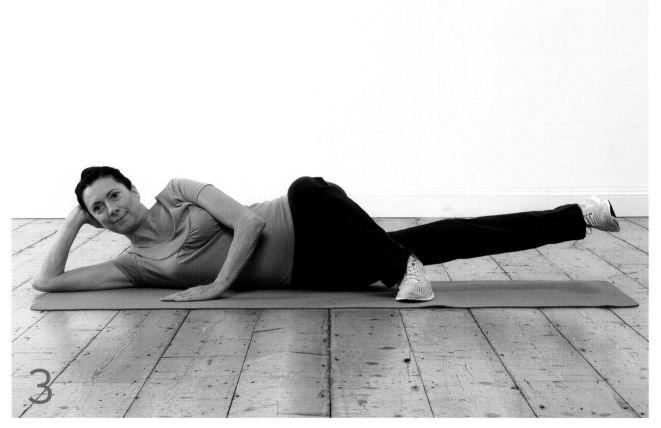

3

Slowly raise your right leg off the floor (you will be able to go higher as you get stronger). Try to keep your leg straight and the toes flexed. Hold for a count of 2, then lower. Aim to do 16 lifts, then repeat on the other side.

Roll-ups

• REPS 20–25
• SETS 1–3

Tightening the oblique muscles of the waist, this exercise also tones your stomach. You may only manage 8 repetitions at first, but should be able to work up to 25 with a little practice.

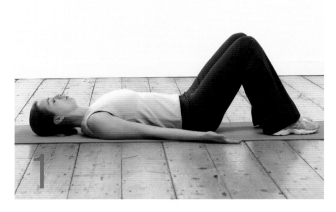

Lie on your back with your knees bent, feet flat on the floor, and hands down by your sides, palms facing up. Pull your stomach muscles toward your spine.

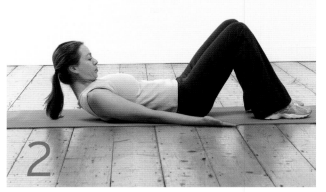

Curl your shoulders and head up and forward, keeping the lower part of your back on the floor.

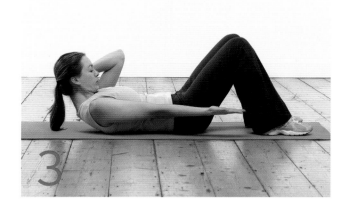

Place your left hand beside your head with the elbow pointing toward your left knee. Lift your right arm off the floor, palm uppermost, keeping your arm low to begin with. As you lift the hand higher toward the knee you will feel your muscles tighten even more at the waist.

WATCHPOINTS

- Keep your lower back flat against the floor and tip your pelvis upward

- Breathe out on the way forward and in on the way back

- Take each movement slowly and focus on the muscles you are working

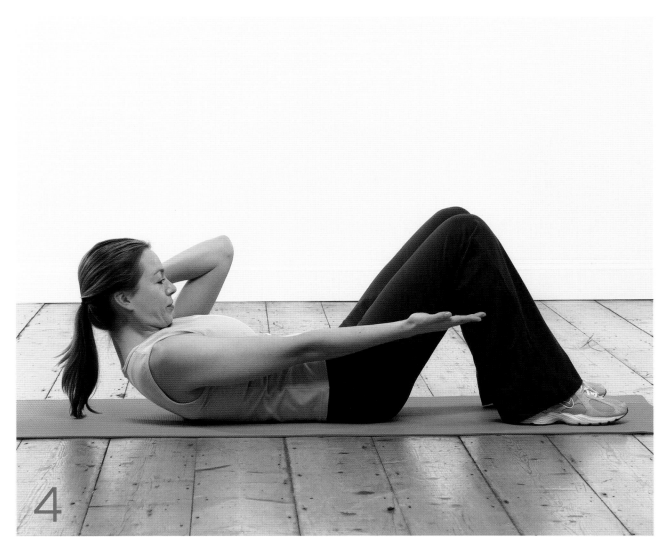

4

Roll forward and up as far as you can, keeping your chin pressed down to your chest, then lower back down to the starting position, but keep your shoulders just off the floor. Without pausing, repeat on the other side.

Bicycle abs

This exercise strengthens the rectus abdominus—the major muscles of the lower stomach. It also helps the external and internal oblique muscles, along with the hip flexors.

1

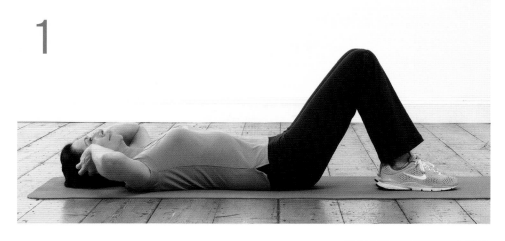

Lying on your back, bend both knees to 90 degrees. Place your hands on each side of your head.

2

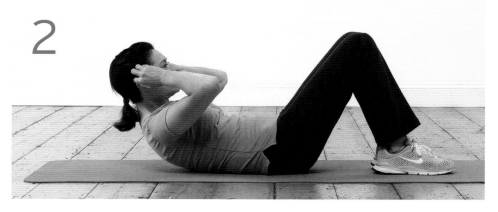

Lift your head and shoulders off the mat.

3

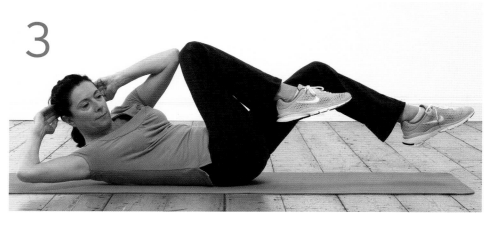

Rotate your legs as if pedaling a bicycle, and move your torso from side to side as you push each elbow to the opposite knee.

WATCHPOINTS

- Make sure there is no stress on your neck

- Breathe out each time your knee comes in to your chest

- Keep your shoulders and head lifted off the floor throughout the exercise

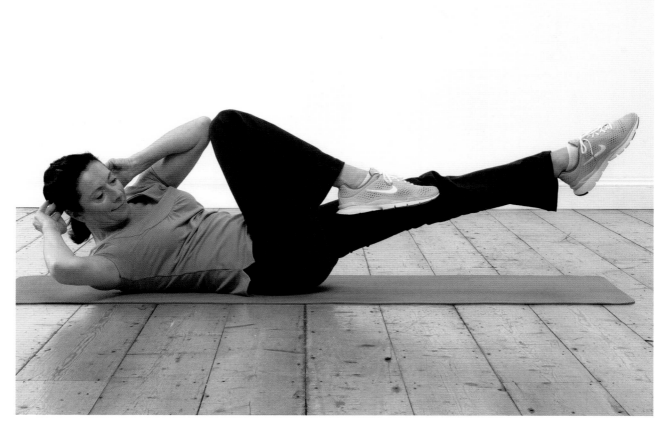

Variation

Try keeping your legs straight as you move them out of each lift.

Crunches

Working on the major stomach muscles, including the external and internal obliques, this exercise will tone and tighten both the front and sides of your stomach.

1

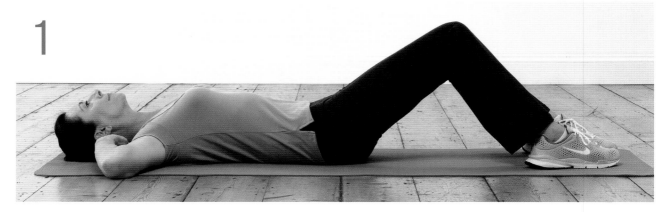

Lie on your back with your knees bent and hip-width apart, feet flat on the floor. Place your hands on each side of your head.

2

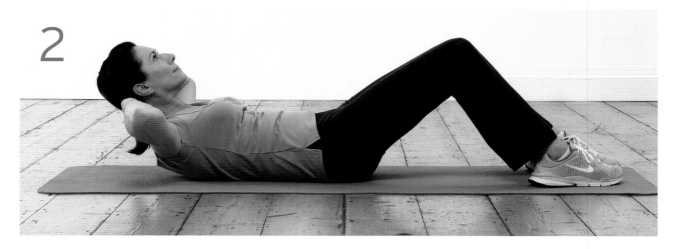

Tighten your stomach muscles and lift your shoulders off the floor, exhaling as you do so. Keep your chin lifted. Hold for a count of 2. Inhale and lower slowly back down, but do not allow your shoulders to touch the floor.

WATCHPOINTS

- The effectiveness of this exercise depends on technique—keep it slow and controlled

- Don't pull on your neck or allow your back to arch

- Make sure both shoulders come off the floor and remain off throughout the exercise

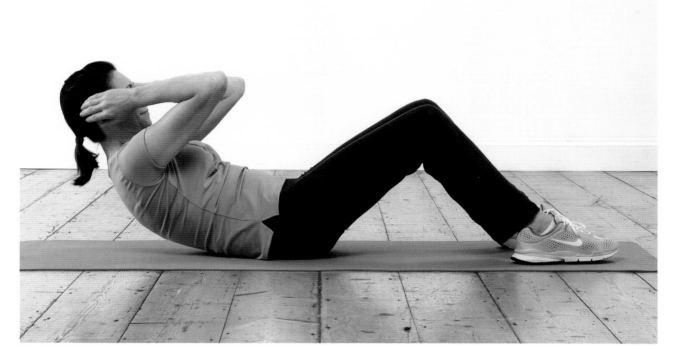

Variation

For a more challenging version of this exercise, continue to curl upward until your shoulders and upper back are lifted off the floor. Hold for a count of 2. Inhale and lower slowly back down, but do not allow your shoulders to touch the floor.

Scissors

This exercise tones the stomach and strengthens the legs, especially the quadriceps muscles and hip flexors. You may only manage a few scissors at first, but this will soon improve.

1

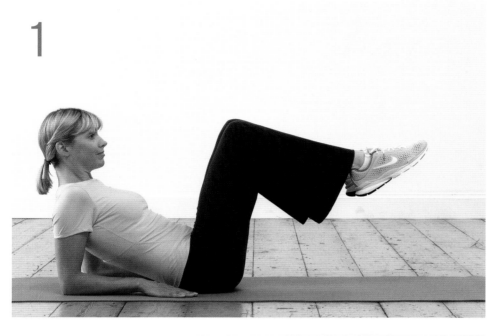

Lying on your back, rest back on your elbows with your hands flat on the floor and fingers pointing toward your bottom. Lean back slightly so your body is at 45 degrees to the floor. Bend your knees and draw them up to your chest.

2

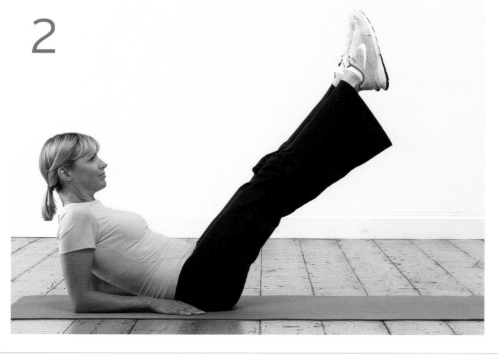

Extend your legs so they are at 45 degrees to the floor. Pull your stomach muscles in and down.

WATCHPOINTS

1 2 3 4 5 6 7 8 9 10 11 12 13

- Don't allow your feet or legs to touch the floor

- There should be no strain through your back

- Keep your stomach tight with the muscles pulled down

3

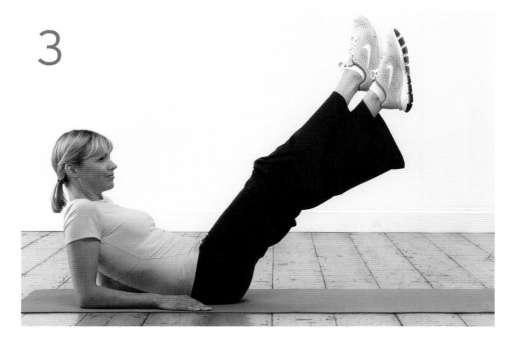

Cross your right leg over your left and then your left leg over your right, moving them in a scissor action.

4

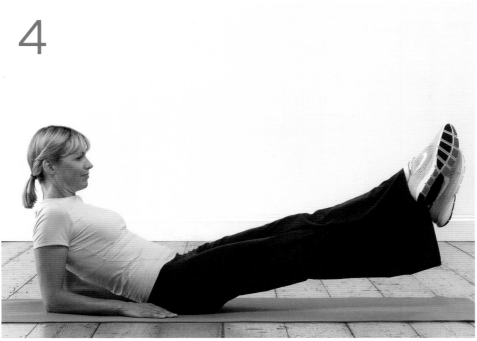

Scissor your legs up and down, taking them as high and as low as you can.

The plank

This exercise is great for strengthening your back, abdomen, and shoulders. It works specifically on the transverse abdominus, the deepest abdominal muscle, to make your waist smaller.

• **REPS 2**
• **SETS 1–3**

WATCHPOINTS

• Maintain your body in a straight line from head to heels

• Keep your hips lifted and your stomach pulled up toward your spine

• Remember to breathe normally as you exercise

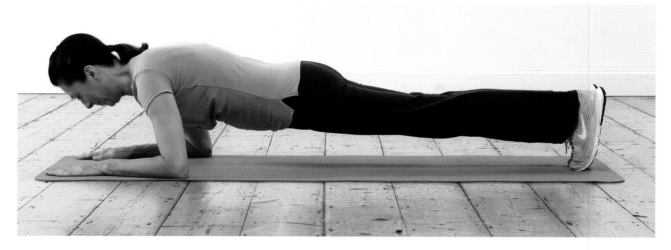

Lie face down with your elbows bent at 90 degrees under your shoulders and your palms and forearms flat on the floor. Push up from the floor, resting on your toes and elbows. Keeping your hips and back in a straight line, pull in your stomach and hold for a count of 20.

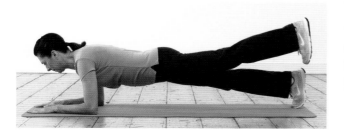

Variation

To increase the intensity of this exercise, lift your left leg straight out behind you and hold. Lower to the original position, then lift your right leg and hold as before.

Side bridge

This exercise targets the abdominals and the external and internal oblique muscles, working your waist and stomach. The longer you hold the lift, the more tension you place on the abdominals.

- **REPS 5–10**
- **SETS 1–3**

WATCHPOINTS

- Pull in your stomach muscles as you lift and keep them tight until you lower back down
- Keep your body in a straight line from shoulders to heels
- Don't let your hips drop

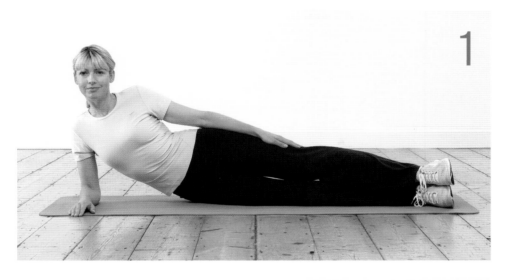

1

Lie on your right side with your body in a straight line and your left leg resting on your right. Rest on your right arm with the elbow bent.

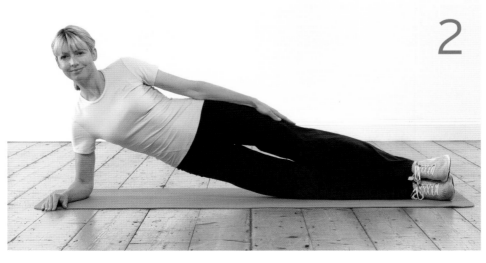

2

Lift your pelvis off the floor, supporting your weight on your right forearm and feet. Your left arm rests on your left leg. Hold for a count of 10, then lower back down. Repeat 5–10 times on each side.

Reverse curls

This exercise will tone and strengthen the major stomach muscles, including the rectus abdominus, and the hip flexors. You may find this a challenging exercise to begin with, but as your muscles strengthen you will be able to do more repetitions.

1

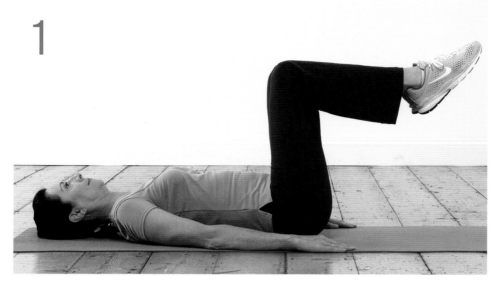

Lie on your back with your knees bent and your feet flat on the floor. Place your arms on each side of your body, resting on the floor. Bend your knees and lift your legs.

2

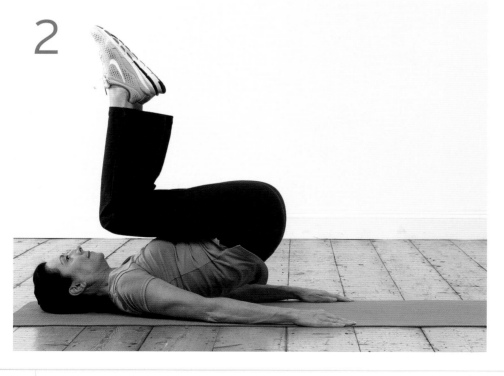

As you tighten your abdominal and stomach muscles, curl your pelvis and legs toward your ribcage, lifting your buttocks off the floor. Keep your legs at 90 degrees to your body. Exhale as you curl up and inhale as you lower back down.

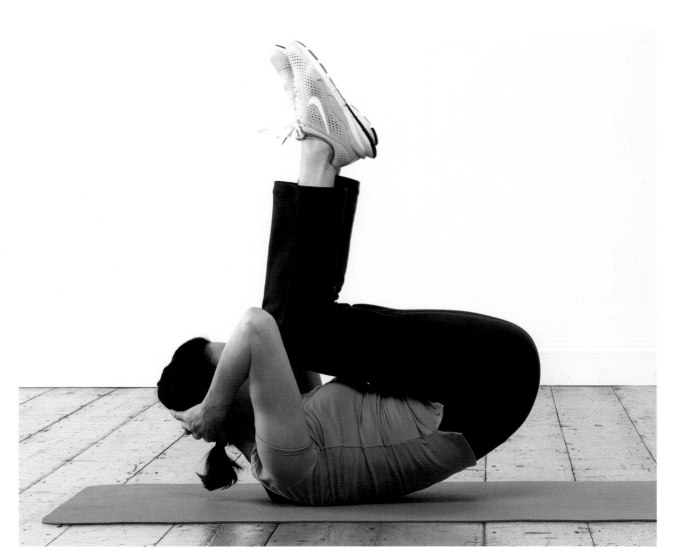

WATCHPOINTS

- Slow, small, controlled movements are required to push your pelvis and lower back off the floor

- If you find this exercise difficult, cross your legs at the ankles

- Don't perform this exercise if you have lower back pain

Variation

To make this exercise more difficult, place your hands on each side of your head and lift your head, neck, and shoulders off the floor at the same time as you lift your buttocks.

Tummy tighteners

• REPS 10–20
• SETS 1–3

Great for tightening the lower abdominal muscles, the hip flexors, and the quadriceps muscles of the thighs, this exercise also strengthens the back's erector spinae and stabilizer muscles.

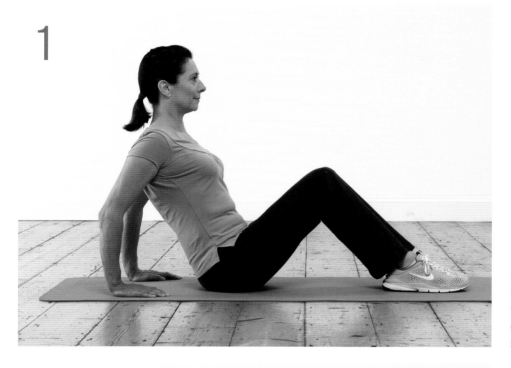

1

Sit with your knees bent, feet flat on the floor and hands resting on the floor on each side of your body.

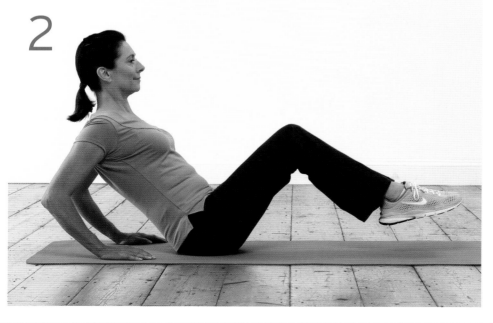

2

Lean back slightly from the hips and lift both legs off the floor, keeping your knees slightly bent and toes pointing down.

WATCHPOINTS

1 2 3 4 5 6 7 8 9 10 11 12 13

- **Keep your chin lifted**

- **There should be no strain through your neck**

- **Keep your stomach muscles pulled in and down**

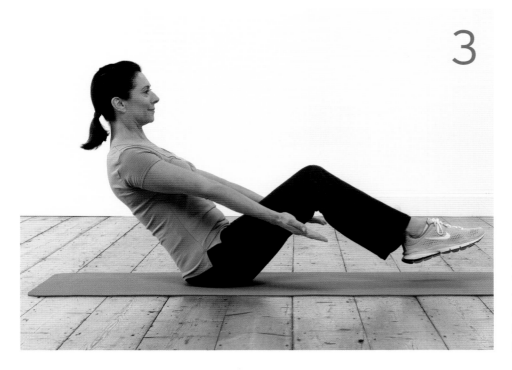

3

Release your arms, stretching them out in front of you, palms facing up. Hold for a count of 4, then lower back down to the starting position.

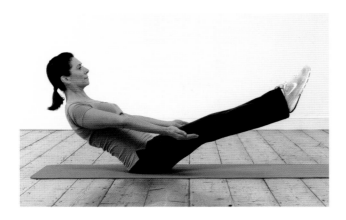

Variation

To increase the intensity of this exercise, straighten your legs and hold.

Oblique crunch

This exercise works the oblique muscles that run down the sides and front of your stomach as well as the upper abdominals. It is often used to target the "love handles" at the sides of the waist.

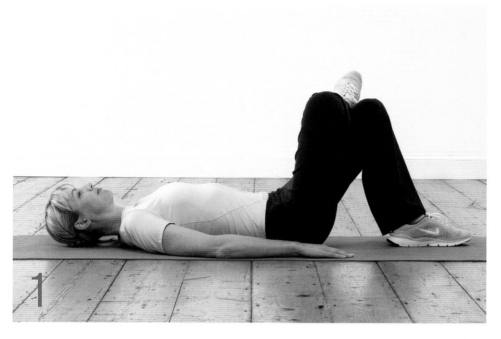

Lie on your back with your knees bent and your left hand at the side of your head. Your right arm and hand rest on the floor. Cross your right leg over your left knee.

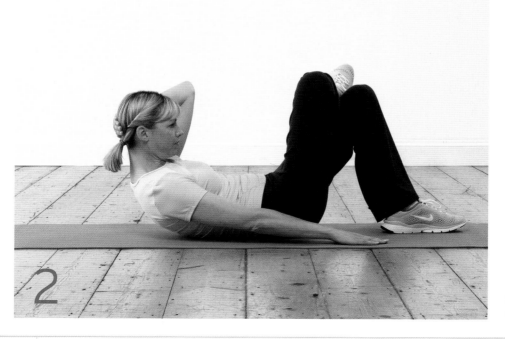

Lift your shoulder blades off the floor, supporting your head with your left hand.

WATCHPOINTS

- Don't thrust your head forward

- Don't pull on the back of your neck with your hands.

- Make sure you use your stomach muscles and not momentum to move

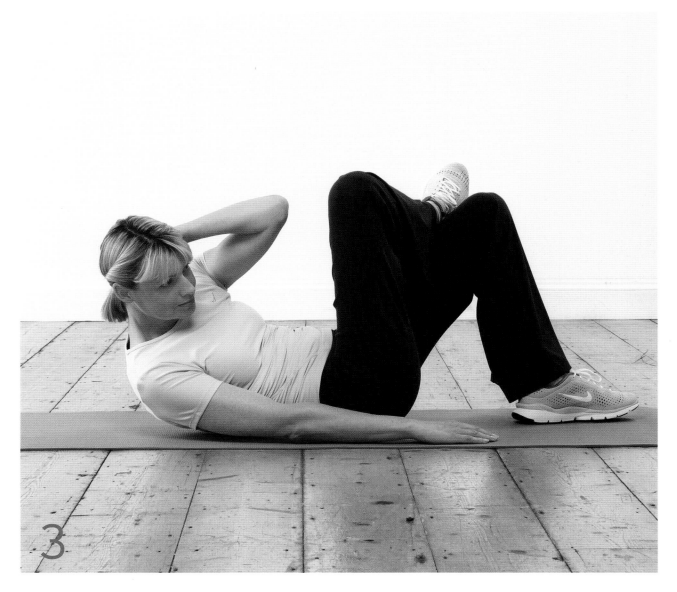

3

Curl your left upper body diagonally across toward your right knee and press your knee away from you. Repeat 10–20 times before changing sides, crossing your left leg over your right knee and lifting your right shoulder.

Double oblique crunch

Although this movement is very similar to the oblique crunch and works the same sets of muscles, it will also strengthen your back muscles and hip flexors.

1

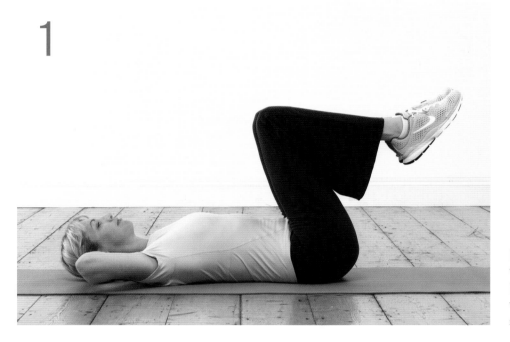

Lie on your back with your knees bent, your legs held in the air, and your hands on each side of your head.

2

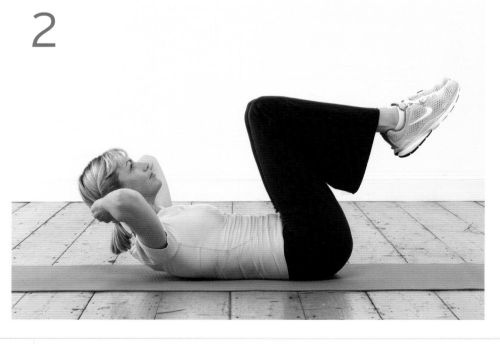

Lift both shoulders up from the floor.

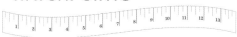

WATCHPOINTS

- Don't pull on your head or neck

- Keep your chin lifted as you crunch your knees in

- Make sure you are breathing correctly

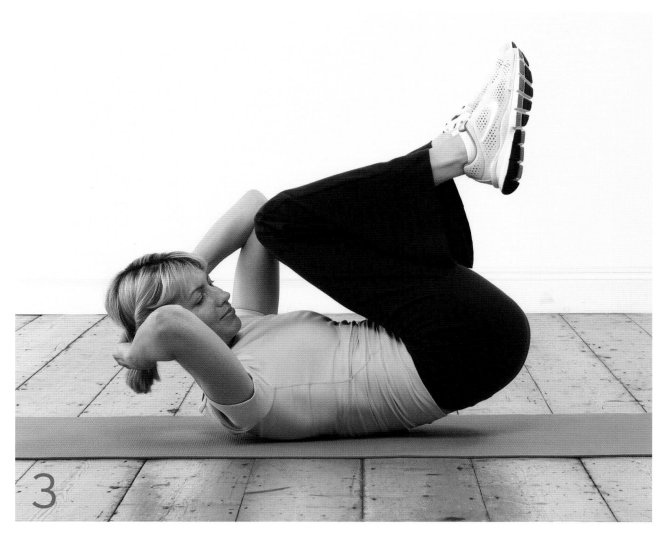

3

Curl your legs and pelvis toward your ribcage, simultaneously curling your shoulders forward. Exhale as you crunch your knees toward your left shoulder. Inhale as you lower back to the starting position. Repeat, bringing your knees in toward your right shoulder. Continue alternating left and right for 10–20 repetitions.

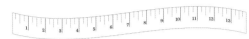

Heel touch

• REPS 10–20
• SETS 1–3

This is another great exercise for working the transverse muscle, the deepest of the stomach muscles and the one that supports the pelvis and lower back. It will help to flatten your stomach.

WATCHPOINTS

- Perform this exercise slowly—it does require good control to maximize its effectiveness

- If you need to make this exercise easier to begin with, bend your leg more and lower it to the floor closer to your buttocks

- Take care not to arch your back during this exercise

1

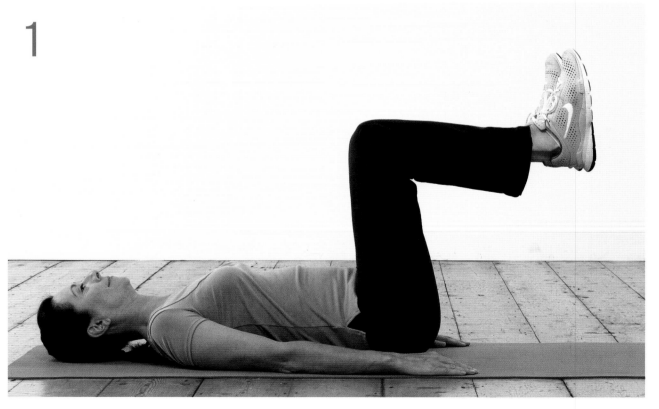

Lie on your back with your knees bent and feet flat on the floor. Place your hands flat on the floor beside your body. Lift your knees until your thighs are at 90 degrees to the floor.

2

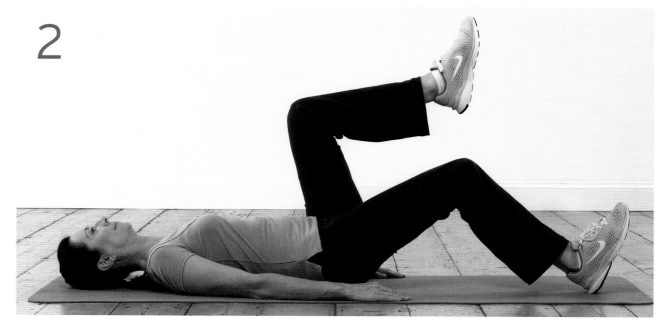

Slowly lower your right leg, keeping your
knee bent, and drop your heel to the floor.

3

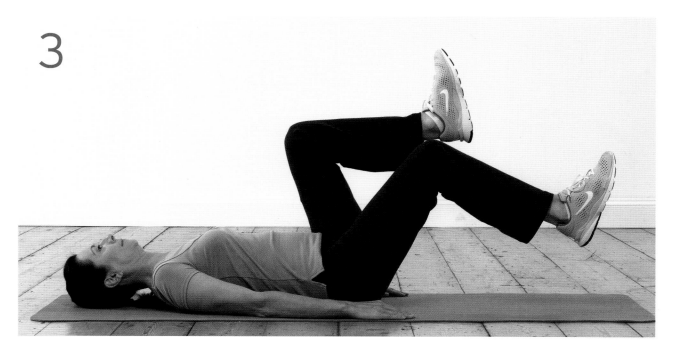

Lift your right leg back up to your chest.
Your left leg remains lifted. Bring your right
knee back, next to your left knee. Repeat
with your left leg.

Extended leg climb

This strong exercise challenges the abdominal muscles, including the rectus abdominus, the obliques, and the hip flexors. Remember to pull your stomach muscles back and down toward your spine.

WATCHPOINTS

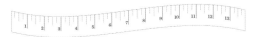

- Keep your elbows soft
- Don't swing your arms to reach forward
- Make sure you are breathing correctly

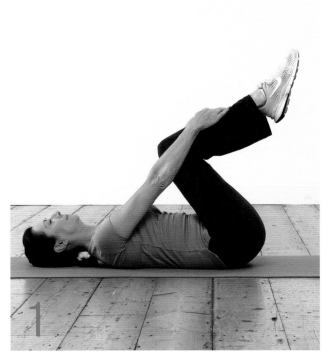

Lie on your back and lift your legs straight up above your hips. Keep your knees slightly bent. Place your hands on your shins while keeping your head and shoulders on the floor.

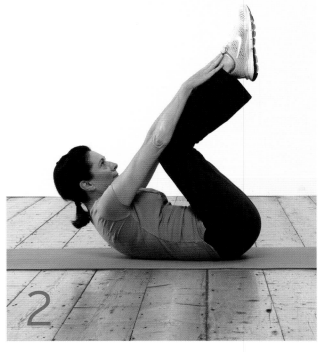

Raise your shoulders off the floor and at the same time move your arms up your shins, then lower back down. Exhale as you lift up and inhale as you lower.

Variation

For a more challenging version of this exercise, move your arms all the way up your shins and straighten your legs with each lift.

Groin stretch

- REPS 1
- SETS 1

This cool-down movement aids flexibility by stretching your groin area, the hip flexors, including the psoas muscle, and the adductor muscles of your inner thighs.

WATCHPOINTS

- Stretch gently, taking care not to bounce

- Push your chest forward, not down, as this keeps your spine long

1

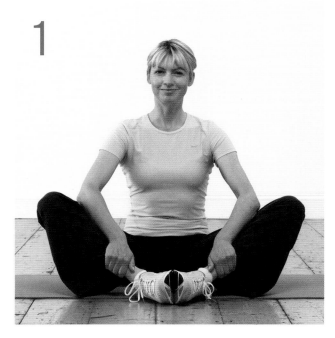

Sit on the floor and put the soles of your feet together. Allow your knees to drop down. Place your hands on top of your feet or around your ankles and your elbows on the insides of your knees.

2

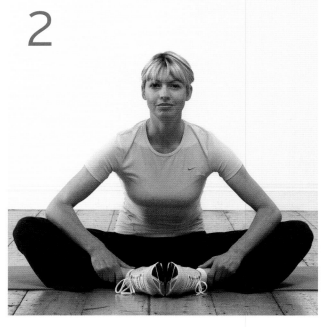

Lean forward from the hips, flattening your back and pressing your knees gently down toward the floor.

Inner thigh stretch

• **REPS 1**
• **SETS 1**

This stretch will run from your groin, through your hip flexors, including the psoas muscle, to the adductor muscles on the inside of your thighs.

WATCHPOINTS

1 2 3 4 5 6 7 8 9 10 11 12 13

• **Keep your upper body straight**

• **Make sure your heels are in a straight line before you begin**

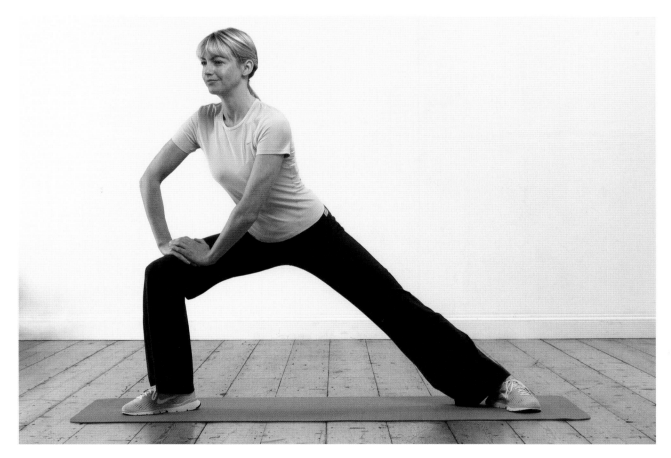

Stand with your feet wide apart. Bend your right knee and take your body weight over to the right. Place both hands on your right thigh. Keep your left leg extended. Hold for a count of 10. Return to the starting position, then repeat to the left side.

Spinal twist

This stretch works your waist and lengthens your spine. It also stretches the hip flexors and the gluteal muscles of your buttocks, and improves posture.

1

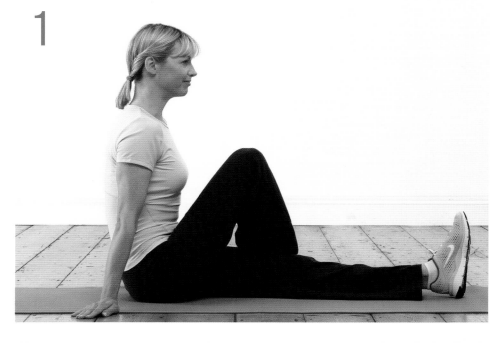

Sit with your legs straight out in front of you. Place your hands flat on the floor on each side of your body. Cross your right leg over your left, bending your right knee and placing your right foot flat on the floor.

2

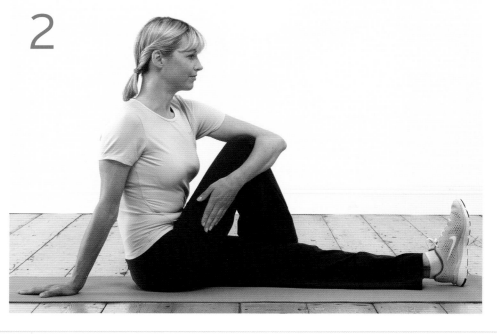

Place your left arm around your right knee so that your fingers and forearm rest on your outer right thigh. Using your left hand, bend your right leg and draw it toward the left side of your body.

WATCHPOINTS

- Keep your spine long and your shoulders relaxed and pulled down

- Exhale as you twist

- Keep your arm wrapped closely around your knee as you hug it to your chest

3

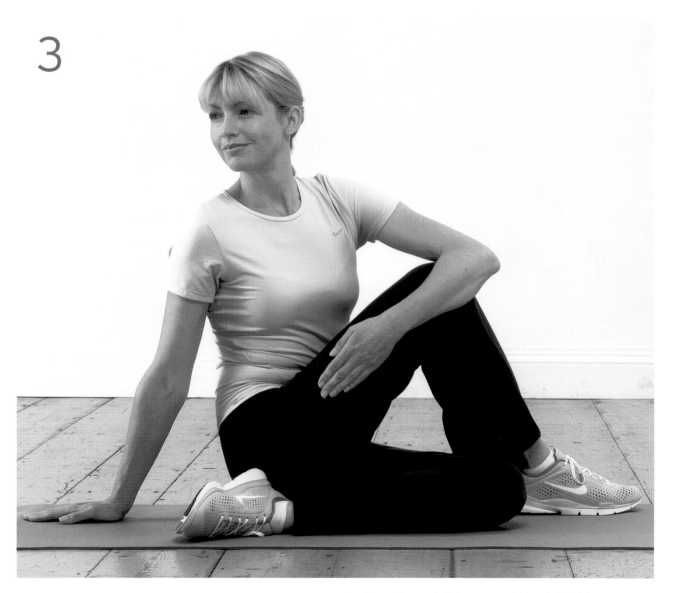

Curl your lower left leg around the right side of your body. Your left heel should be close to your right buttock. Turn your head and look over your right shoulder. Hold for a count of 5. Return to the starting position and repeat to the other side.

Pose of the child

• **REPS 1**
• **SETS 1**

This is a relaxation exercise as well as a stretch. You will feel the stretch through the spinal muscles, easing tension in your back, thighs, and hips.

1

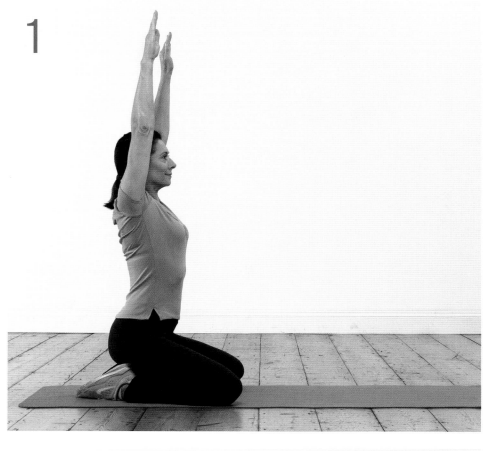

Kneel and sit back on your heels. Open your knees wide and lift both arms straight up to the ceiling.

2

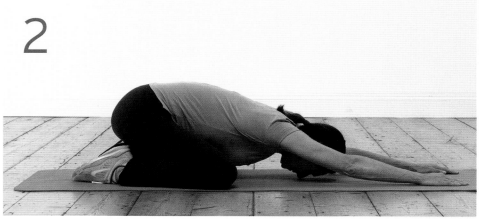

Lower your chest and arms to the floor, with your buttocks remaining on your heels. Stretch forward and hold for a count of 10. Lift your arms back up toward the ceiling, raising your chest to the starting position.

WATCHPOINTS

- Do not perform this exercise if you have any knee problems. However, the exercise can be used to relieve back pain.

- Breathe in and out gently as you remain in the lowered position.

- Inhale as you come back up to a sitting position.

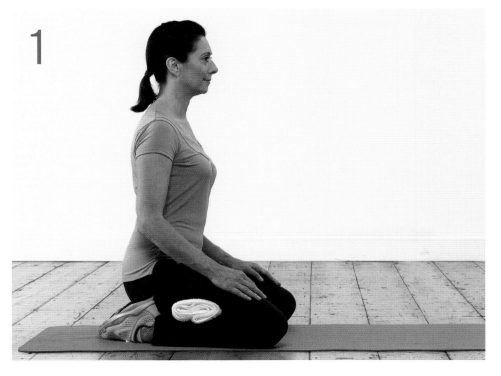

Variation

Some people may be more comfortable using a towel to sit on during this stretch. Kneel as before, inserting a rolled-up towel behind your knees.

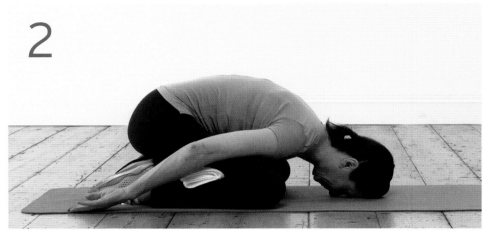

An easier variation is to stretch out your arms behind you as you lower your chest to the floor, holding for a count of 5.

Index

A

abdominal fat 8, 11
abdominal muscles *see* stomach
    muscles
adipose tissue 15
adrenal glands 12, 17, 18
adrenalin 12–13
aerobic exercise 72, 74
aging 13
alcohol 25, 27
almonds: almondy angel cakes 65
  baked pear with almond crumble 47
alpha linoleic fatty acid 15
angina 8
angler fish with asparagus 65
antioxidants 18
appetite 11, 12, 13
"apple shape" body 8, 11
apples: baked apples 59
  carrot and apple juice 40
arabesque 90–1
arm exercises: lunges with lateral
    raises 92–3
  upper body warm-up 77
arteriosclerosis 8
artichoke hearts: griddled artichokes
    and fennel 47
  ricotta, smoked salmon, and
    artichoke wrap 35
asparagus 18
  angler fish with asparagus 65
aubergines with chili toasts 59
avocados 18, 44
  avocado and sunflower seed
    salad 64
  avocado open sandwich 58
  crudités with guacamole 56

B

back exercises: double oblique
    crunch 112–13
  the plank 104
  pose of the child 122–3
  spinal twist 120–1

tummy tighteners 108–9
back pain 9
bagels, savory 38, 52
bananas: baked bananas 39
  banana smoothie 68
  mango and banana smoothie 30
  strawberry and banana
    smoothie 44
beans 30
  bean and feta stir-fry 65
  bean and lamb roast 57
  bean curry 30
  chicken and bean salad 46
  vegetable and bean soup 54
  vegetarian chili 61
beef: peppered steak 35
  steak and mixed rice 69
berries 18, 62
bicycle abs 98–9
blood pressure 8, 9
blood sugar levels 7, 13, 16
body fat 11, 13
  excess glucose stored as 16
  waist-to-hip ratio (WHR) 11
Body Mass Index (BMI) 8, 10–11
body shape 8, 11
bones, osteoporosis 9
bottom lifts 87
breast cancer 9
bridge, side 105
broccoli, pasta with olives,
    mozzarella, and 55
bulgar wheat salad 40
buttock exercises: bottom lifts 87
  buttock kicks 86
  side leg lifts 89
  spinal twist 120–1

C

cabbage 18
cakes, almondy angel 65
calcium 18
calf stretch 80
calories: and body fat percentage 13
  counting 16
  metabolism and 18, 19
  reducing fat 15
  weight gain 11

cancer 9
capsaicin 18, 68
carbohydrates 14
  boosting metabolism 18
  controlling insulin production 18
  cravings 13
  glycaemic index 16
  regulating hormones 17
carotenoids 18
carrot and apple juice 40
cauliflower cheese soup 56
celery 18
cheese: bean and feta stir-fry 65
  cauliflower cheese soup 56
  cottage cheese and herb
    sandwich 60
  cottage cheese and salad 62
  feta salad 50
  griddled artichokes and fennel 47
  pasta with broccoli, olives, and
    mozzarella 55
  whole-wheat pita with cottage
    cheese 52
chicken: broiled chicken 45
  chicken and bean salad 46
  chicken and rice salad 56
  chicken salad Thai style 39
  flaming chicken 49
  ginger baked chicken 63
  Jamaican chicken with sweet
    potato wedges 31
  spiced chicken and pearl barley 61
chicken liver salad 67
chickpeas: chickpea and olive
    salad 38
  oven-baked crunchy chickpeas 36
chili, vegetarian 61
chocolate 13
cholesterol 8, 15
chromium 17, 18
clothing, for exercise 74
cod: cod and roasted
    vegetables 59
  Spanish fish stew 37
coffee 25
colon cancer 9
cool-down exercises 74
cortisol 9, 12–13, 17

couscous, fruity 43
cravings 7, 13, 24
crêpes: ricotta, smoked salmon, and
    artichoke wrap 35
crunches 100–1
    double oblique crunch 112–13
    oblique crunch 110–11
cucumber: raita 61
curls, reverse 106–7
curry, bean 30

D E
dehydration 18, 25, 74
depression 34
diabetes 8, 9, 12
diet see food
"diet" foods 16
dinner 24–5
double oblique crunch 112–13
drinks 18, 25, 74
eggs 54
    see also omelets
essential fatty acids (EFAs) 15, 17
exercise: aerobic exercise 72, 74
    benefits of 9, 72
    metabolism and 13, 72
    planning 21
    reps and sets 74
    Waistline Exercise plan, 70–123
extended leg climb 116–17

F
fatigue 9
fats, in diet 15
    see also body fat
fennel, griddled artichokes
    and 47
fertility problems 9
fiber 14, 18
figs, honeyed 31
flax seeds 32
flounder parcels 69
food: boosting metabolism 18–19
    diet maintenance plan 27
    failed diets 7
    fighting pollution with 18
    foods to avoid 26
    nutrition 14–16

regulating hormones with 17–18
    shopping list 20–1, 26
    Waistline Diet plan 22–69
free radicals 18
fruit 18, 25
    exotic fruit salad 54
    fresh fruit compote 38
    fruit smoothie 48, 56, 60

G
gallbladder disease 9
ghrelin 12, 13
ginger baked chicken 63
glucose: diabetes 8
    glycaemic index 16
    insulin and 12
glycaemic index 16
goals 20
granola 34, 40, 50, 56
groin stretch 118
guacamole, crudités with 56

H
halibut, broiled 43
ham and mushroom
    omelet 62
hamstring stretch 81
HDL cholesterol 15
health risks, overweight 8–9
heart disease 8, 9
heel touch 114–15
herby lamb 41
hip exercises: groin stretch 118
    inner thigh stretch 119
    pose of the child 122–3
    spinal twist 120–1
honeyed figs 31
hormones: appetite control 11, 12
    exercise and 9
    lack of sleep and 13
    and middle-age spread 12
    regulating with food 17–18
    stress and 12–13
hummus, vegetable crudités with
    34, 44
hunger 12, 16, 60
hydrogenated fats 15
hypertension 8

I J
infertility 9
inner thigh lifts 94–5
inner thigh stretch 119
insulin 12
    controlling production of 18
    diabetes 8
    and glucose consumption 16
    insulin resistance 9, 11, 12, 13
    and weight gain 12, 17
Jamaican chicken with sweet potato
    wedges 31
joints, osteoarthritis 9

K L
kebabs, vegetable 28
knee lifts 83
lamb: bean and lamb roast 57
    herby lamb 41
LDL cholesterol 8, 15
leg exercises: arabesque 90–1
    buttock kicks 86
    calf stretch 80
    extended leg climb 116–17
    groin stretch 118
    hamstring stretch 81
    heel touch 114–15
    inner thigh lifts 94–5
    inner thigh stretch 119
    knee lifts 83
    leg lifts 88
    lunges with lateral raises 92–3
    quads stretch 82
    scissors 102–3
    side leg lifts 89
    squat jumps 85
    squats 84
    tummy tighteners 108–9
legumes 30
lentils: lentil pilaff 41
    red lentil dhal 31
    scallops in pancetta with lemon
    lentils 51
leptin 11, 12, 13, 18
lima beans, tangy 41
linoleic fatty acid 15
lipoproteins 8, 15
liver, visceral fat and 11

low-calorie foods 16
lunges with lateral raises 92–3

M
mangoes: mango and banana
    smoothie 30
    mango sorbet 69
Mediterranean peppers 37
melon, oriental 49
menopause 11, 12, 13
menus 28–69
metabolism: boosting 18–19
    exercise and 13, 72
    muscles and 13
    "yo-yo" dieting 7
middle-age spread: causes of 12–13
    health risks 8–9
milk thistle 18
minerals 14
miso broth 36
monounsaturated fat 15
motivation 21
muscles 13, 73, 75
mushrooms: ham and mushroom
    omelet 62
    mushroom stroganoff 33
mussels: Spanish fish stew 37

N O
noodles: stir-fried noodles 39
    vegetable noodles 49
nutrition see food
nuts 42
oats 66
    crunchy yogurt 52, 66
    porridge 28
oblique crunch 110–11
    double oblique crunch 112–13
oestrogen 11, 13, 15, 30
olives, pasta with broccoli,
    mozzarella, and 55
omega-3 oils 15, 18
omega-6 oils 15
omelets: ham and mushroom
    omelet 62
    omelet and salad 32
    savory omelet 54, 68
    vegetable omelet 48

oranges: radicchio and orange
    salad 69
oriental melon 49
osteoarthritis 9
osteoporosis 9

P
pancetta, scallops in 51
pasta: pasta with broccoli, olives, and
    mozzarella 55
    roast pepper and walnut
        pappardelle 45
    vegetable penne 67
peaches, baked 55
"pear shape" body 11
pearl barley, spiced chicken and 61
pears: baked pear with almond
    crumble 47
peppered steak 35
peppers 18, 68
    Mediterranean peppers 37
    roast pepper and walnut
        pappardelle 45
perimenopause 12, 13
phytochemicals 18
phytoestrogens 30
pilaff, lentil 41
pineapple 51
    broiled pineapple and plum
        sauce 37
pita: whole-wheat pita with cottage
    cheese 52
    whole-wheat pita with turkey
        salad 34
    whole-wheat tuna pita 40
the plank 104
planning 20–1
plums: broiled pineapple and plum
    sauce 37
pollution 13, 18
polyunsaturated fat 15
pomegranates 38
porridge 28
pose of the child 122–3
protein 14, 17, 18

Q R
quads stretch 82

quinoa and rice fluff 53
radicchio and orange salad 69
raita 61
raspberries: strawberry and
    raspberry smoothie 36
reps, exercises 74
restaurants 40
reverse curls 106–7
rice 18
    chicken and rice salad 56
    mixed rice and vegetables 48
    quinoa and rice fluff 53
    rice salad 66
    steak and mixed rice 69
ricotta, smoked salmon, and
    artichoke wrap 35
roll-ups 96–7

S
safety, exercise 74
salads: avocado and sunflower seed
    salad 64
    bulgar wheat salad 40
    chicken and bean salad 46
    chicken and rice salad 56
    chicken salad Thai style 39
    chickpea and olive salad 38
    cottage cheese and salad 62
    feta salad 50
    hot chicken liver salad 67
    radicchio and orange salad 69
    rice salad 66
    tuna salad 50, 68
    whole-wheat pita with turkey
        salad 34
salmon fillet, baked 55
salsa, lemony 29
sandwiches: avocado open
    sandwich 58
    cottage cheese and herb
        sandwich 60
    wholegrain turkey sandwich 50
saturated fat 15
scallops in pancetta with lemon
    lentils 51
scissors exercise 102–3
sea bass, broiled 33
selenium 18

serotonin 13, 34
sesame seeds 18
sets, exercises 74
shopping list 20–1, 26
shoulder exercises, the plank 104
shrimp: marinated shrimp with
    zucchini 53
  shrimp stir-fry 57
  shrimp tortilla 64
side bridge 105
side leg lifts 89
side twist 79
sleep, lack of 13
sleep apnoea 9
smoked salmon, ricotta, and
    artichoke wrap 35
smoothies: banana smoothie 68
  fruit smoothie 48, 56, 60
  mango and banana smoothie 30
  strawberry and banana
    smoothie 44
  strawberry and raspberry
    smoothie 36
snacks 25
somatopause 8
sorbet, mango 69
soups: cauliflower cheese soup 56
  miso broth 36
  vegetable and bean soup 54
  watercress soup 32
Spanish fish stew 37
spinal twist 120–1
spring rolls, Vietnamese
    vegetable 43
squat jumps 85
squats 84
starchy foods 14
starvation, "yo-yo" dieting 7
steak and mixed rice 69
steps 76
stomach muscles: and back pain 9
  bicycle abs 98–9
  crunches 100–1
  double oblique crunch 112–13
  extended leg climb 116–17
  heel touch 114–15
  oblique crunch 110–11
  the plank 104

reverse curls 106–7
roll-ups 96–7
scissors 102–3
side bridge 105
tummy tighteners 108–9
strawberries: strawberries and
    yogurt 57
  strawberry and banana
    smoothie 44
  strawberry and raspberry
    smoothie 36
  strawberry whip 45
stress 7, 12–13, 18
stretching exercises: arm
    stretches 77
  calf stretch 80
  groin stretch 118
  hamstring stretch 81
  inner thigh stretch 119
  pose of the child 122–3
  quads stretch 82
  side stretch 78
stroke 8, 9
subcutaneous fat 11
sugar 13, 14, 16
sunflower seeds 18
  avocado and sunflower seed
    salad 64
sunlight, as appetite suppressant 12
sweet potato wedges, Jamaican
    chicken with 31

T
tea 25
  green tea 18
thighs see legs
tiredness 9
tofu: sizzling tofu 35
  tofu and roasted vegetables 59
  tofu with vegetables 63
tomatoes 46
  Spanish fish stew 37
tortillas 30
  shrimp tortilla 64
trans fats 15
triglycerides 8
trout, baked 67
tummy tighteners 108–9

tuna: seared tuna with lemony
    salsa 29
  tuna salad 50, 68
  whole-wheat tuna pita 40
turkey: wholegrain turkey
    sandwich 50
  whole-wheat pita with turkey
    salad 34
twisting exercises: side twist 79
  spinal twist 120–1

V
vegetables 18, 25
  cod and roasted vegetables 59
  crudités with guacamole 56
  crudités with hummus 34, 44
  spicy vegetable roast 63
  tofu with vegetables 63
  vegetable and bean soup 54
  vegetable kebabs 28
  vegetable noodles 49
  vegetable penne 67
  Vietnamese vegetable spring
    rolls 43
vegetarian chili 61
Vietnamese vegetable spring rolls 43
vitamins 14, 15, 17, 18

W Y Z
waist circumference 11
waist-to-hip ratio (WHR) 11
Waistline Diet plan 22–69
Waistline Exercise plan, 70–123
warm-up exercises 74
water, drinking 18, 25, 74
watercress soup 32
weight: Body Mass Index (BMI)
    8, 10–11
  diet maintenance plan 27
weights, hand 74
wholegrains 58
"yo-yo" dieting 7
yogurt: crunchy yogurt 52, 66
  raita 61
  strawberries and yogurt 57
zinc 17
zucchini, marinated shrimp
    with 53

Acknowledgments

AUTHOR ACKNOWLEDGMENTS

I would like to thank Jane and her team at Hamlyn.
Also, my sons, Alex and Harrison, Mum and Dad for their
continued support, Fiona for her culinary expertise, and,
of course, Mark, for his inspiration.

PUBLISHER ACKNOWLEDGMENTS

Executive editor Jane McIntosh
Editor Fiona Robertson
Executive art editor Karen Sawyer
Designer Martin Topping
Senior production controller Manjit Sihra
Picture library Sophie Delpech
Picture research Aruna Mathur

PICTURE ACKNOWLEDGMENTS

Special Photography © **Octopus Publishing Group
Limited**/Mike Prior.

Alamy 36. **Corbis UK Limited**/LWA-Dann Tardif 13;
/George Shelley 8. **Getty Images** 21; /Brooke Fasani 6;
/Deborah Jaffe 9. **Octopus Publishing Group Limited**/
Frank Adam 14 center left, 14 bottom right, 18 left, 34, 52,
68; /Stephen Conroy 33, 35, 37, 43, 47, 49, 62, 63, 64, 65;
/Jeremy Hopley 40; /David Jordan 17 bottom; /Sandra
Lane 14 top left, 44; /William Lingwood 14 center right,
15, 28, 30, 46, 48, 66; /Peter Myers 17 top; /Sean Myers
14 bottom left; /Ian O'Leary 19; /Lis Parsons 29, 31, 39, 41,
45, 51, 53, 55, 57, 58, 59, 61, 67, 69; /Peter Pugh-Cook 75
bottom; /William Reavell 16, 32, 42; /Gareth Sambidge 18
right, 27, 50, 56; /Simon Smith 14 top right; /Ian Wallace
38, 54, 60. **Photolibrary** 74.